Colour **Aids**

Orthopaedics

Geoffrey Hooper MMSc FRCS FRCS(Ed)

Senior Lecturer in Orthopaedic Surgery,
University of Edinburgh; Honorary
Consultant Orthopaedic Surgeon, Royal
Infirmary and Princess Margaret Rose
Orthopaedic Hospital, Edinburgh, and
Bangour General Hospital, West Lothian, UK

Churchill Livingstone

EDINBURGH LONDON MELBOURNE AND NEW YORK 1986

CHURCHILL LIVINGSTONE
Medical Division of Longman Group Limited

Distributed in the United States of America by
Churchill Livingstone Inc., 1560 Broadway, New
York, N.Y. 10036, and by associated companies,
branches and representatives throughout the
world.

First published 1986

ISBN 0-443-03292-0

British Library Cataloguing in Publication Data
Hooper, Geoffrey
 Orthopaedics.—(Colour aids)
 1. Orthopedia—Atlases
 I. Title   II. Series
 617'.3'00222   RD733.2

Library of Congress Cataloging in Publication Data
Hooper, Geoffrey.
 Orthopaedics.
 (Colour aids)
 1. Orthopedia—Atlases.   I. Title.   II. Series.
[DNLM: 1. Orthopedics—atlases.   WE 17 H7860]
RD733.2.H66   1985   617'.3   85-14929

Produced by Longman Group (FE) Ltd.
Printed in Hong Kong

Acknowledgements

I thank the following colleagues who have generously provided illustrations: Mr J. Chalmers (Figs 80, 81, 82, 87); Professor P. J. Gregg (Figs 45, 47, 67, 79, 163, 167, 182, 191); Professor S. P. F. Hughes (Figs 2, 23, 50, 51, 53, 56, 76, 77, 101, 120, 172, 177, 203, 204); Mr M. R. H. Khan (Figs 40, 41, 42); Mr D. W. Lamb (Figs 133, 135, 136, 137); Mr M. J. McMaster (Figs 24, 104); Mr M. F. Macnicol (Figs 32, 33, 74, 155); Professor G. Nuki (Fig. 34); Mr J. Phillips (Fig. 7); Mr J. H. S. Scott (Figs 112, 113).

I am also grateful to Professor Hughes for allowing me to use slides from the collection in the Department of Orthopaedic Surgery, University of Edinburgh (Figs 1, 16, 31, 35, 36, 37, 46, 52, 59, 60, 61, 75, 92, 95, 98, 100, 103, 130, 176, 190, 195).

I thank Michael Devlin and Avril Nesbit for their assistance in the preparation of photographic material and Alison McGowan for her careful typing of the manuscript.

Contents

1 | Infections (1)

Acute osteomyelitis

Infection of bone due to pyogenic bacteria (usually staphylocoici or streptococci).

Pathology

Bacteria may enter the bone directly, e.g. from an open fracture, or via the blood stream from a septic focus elsewhere in the body. In the latter (haematogenous) type of osteomyelitis the infection usually begins in the metaphysis of a long bone. If untreated, infection may cause thrombosis of blood vessels and death of bone. An abscess may form under the periosteum and then burst into surrounding soft tissues.

Clinical features

Haematogenous osteomyelitis usually affects children. There is a fairly rapid onset with malaise, pyrexia and pain over the affected part. Examination reveals local tenderness, warmth and often erythema (Fig. 1).

Investigations

Radiographs negative in the early stage, but later a subperiosteal reaction may be seen (Fig. 2). An isotope bone scan is positive at an early stage (Fig. 3).
ESR is raised.
The infecting organism may be identified by culturing blood withdrawn before antibiotics are started.

Treatment

Early stage. Rest. Broad spectrum antibiotics in high dosage pending identification of the organism.
Later stage. Surgical drainage is necessary if there is no response to appropriate antibiotic therapy, or if an abscess has formed.

Complications

Septicaemia, chronic osteomyelitis, and septic arthritis (p. 3), damage to growth plate causing deformity in growing bone.

GENERAL ORTHOPAEDICS

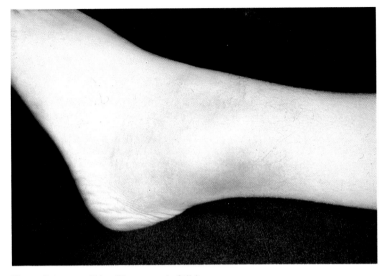

Fig. 1 Osteomyelitis of lower end of tibia.

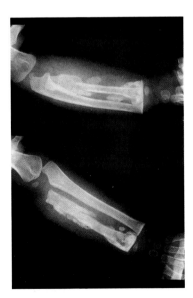

Fig. 2 Untreated acute osteomyelitis of the radius, showing vigorous periosteal reaction.

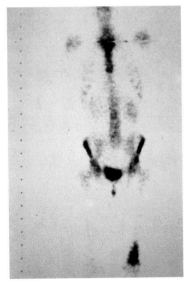

Fig. 3 Bone scan showing increased uptake at the lower end of the left femur.

| **Infections (2)**

Chronic osteomyelitis

Chronic infection of bone that usually follows an attack of acute osteomyelitis that has not been treated adequately.

Pathology

The bone is thickened and filled with granulation tissue. Sinuses lead from the bone to the skin surface (Fig. 4). Pieces of dead bone (sequestra) are sometimes visible on radiographs (Fig. 5).

Clinical features

Pain, intermittent discharge of pus from sinuses.

Treatment

Very difficult. Appropriate antibiotics will control flare-ups of infection. Surgical removal of a sequestrum may allow a sinus to heal, but for permanent cure all dead and infected material must be removed.

Septic arthritis

Bacterial infection of a joint, usually by the pyogenic organisms associated with acute osteomyelitis. Organisms can enter the joint by the haematogenous route, by direct entry through a wound or from adjacent infected bone. The latter route is important if the infected metaphysis of a long bone lies within the joint capsule (e.g. proximal metaphyses of humerus and femur).

Clinical features

Pyrexia and malaise. Affected joint is swollen, tender and warm. Radiographs are normal at first, later show periarticular osteoporosis and then joint destruction (Fig. 6).

Treatment

Rest, splintage and antibiotics. Surgical drainage, rather than aspiration, is usually necessary and should be done early since, once damaged, articular cartilage does not regenerate.

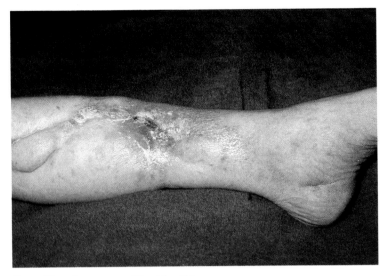

Fig. 4 Chronic osteomyelitis of the tibia.

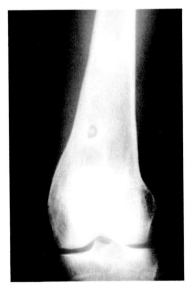

Fig. 5 A small sequestrum within the lower part of the femur.

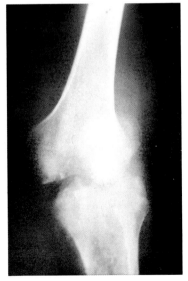

Fig. 6 Gross destruction of the knee joint due to septic arthritis in a diabetic patient.

1 | Infections (3)

Tuberculosis

Bones and joints can be infected by one of the various types of tubercle bacilli. Infection can occur at any age. The tubercle bacilli enter bone via the blood stream or by direct spread from another focus.

Clinical features

The patient is usually unwell with the general signs of tuberculosis, e.g. weight loss, pyrexia, night sweats.
Specific features depend on the joint involved. Large joints and the spine are most often affected but small bones in the hand can be involved (dactylitis).
Large joints. There is pain, swelling and limitation of movement; the muscles around the joints are often wasted.
Spine. Destruction of the intervertebral disc and adjacent vertebrae may cause a kyphosis (Fig. 7). Paraplegia may be a feature. Infected material may track downwards and form an abscess in the groin (a psoas abscess).

Investigations

Radiographs show destruction of joints (Fig. 9) and a paravertebral abscess may be seen in the spine (Fig. 8). Mantoux test is positive.
ESR is raised in the active phase.
A biopsy of the affected area will show the histological features of tuberculosis.

Treatment

Rest and splintage of affected joint.
Antituberculous chemotherapy. Arthrodesis of painful, unstable joints. Surgical drainage and stabilisation of spinal lesions may be indicated, particularly if there are neurological signs or an increasing kyphosis.

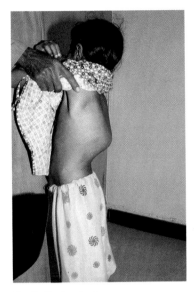

Fig. 7 Kyphosis due to tuberculous infection of spine.

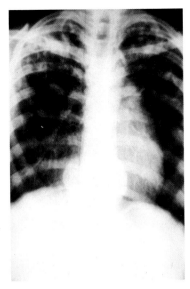

Fig. 8 Paravertebral abscess seen behind heart shadow.

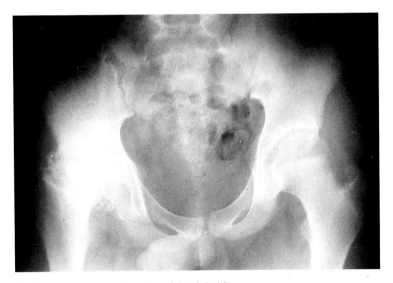

Fig. 9 Tuberculous destruction of the right hip.

2 | Arthritis (1)

Osteoarthritis (degenerative arthritis; osteoarthrosis)

A common condition which is due to 'wear and tear' of joints.
It may be primary (idiopathic) or secondary to any condition that causes damage or irregularity of the joint surface, such as injury, avascular necrosis (p. 47), osteochondritis dissecans (p. 127) and septic arthritis (p. 3).

Clinical features

More common with advancing age.
One major weight bearing joint such as the hip is usually affected in secondary osteoarthritis (OA) but primary OA may affect several joints. The joints affected are painful and stiff and may become deformed.

Investigations

Radiographs show loss of joint space, sclerosis of subchondral bone, osteophytes and cysts (Fig. 10), although all these features may not be present.

Treatment

Analgesics.
Physiotherapy is symptomatically helpful in many cases.
Obese patients should lose weight. Surgical treatment may be indicated if these general measures are unhelpful. Procedures that may be considered are:
Arthrodesis.　Surgical fusion of a joint (Fig. 11). Most often indicated for small joints as arthrodesis of large joints such as hip or knee may be disabling despite relief of pain.
Osteotomy.　Realignment of a joint by cutting through adjacent bone (Fig. 12). Effective in correcting deformity but pain relief is unpredictable.
Excision arthroplasty.　Surgical removal of a joint (Fig. 13). Seldom used as a primary treatment for OA in large joints.
Replacement arthroplasty.　See p. 9.

GENERAL ORTHOPAEDICS

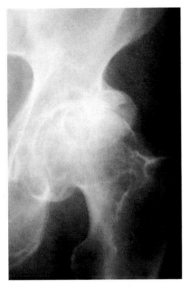

Fig. 10 Osteoarthritis of the hip.

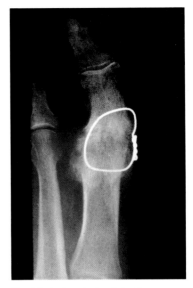

Fig. 11 Arthrodesis of the first metatarsophalangeal joint.

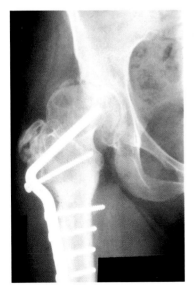

Fig. 12 Valgising upper femoral osteotomy for OA of the hip.

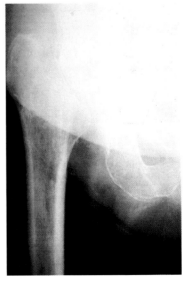

Fig. 13 Excision arthroplasty of the hip (Girdlestone arthroplasty).

Osteoarthritis (contd)

Treatment

Total joint replacement for joints affected by OA, particularly the hip, has become the most common major orthopaedic procedure. Artificial replacements have been designed for many joints; they have been most successful in the hip but have not yet come into wide use in other joints affected by OA. An artificial joint consists of metal and high density polyethylene components (Fig. 14). These materials are used because of their generally satisfactory frictional and wear characteristics. The components are stabilised in position with methylmethacrylate cement (Fig. 15).

Complications

A successful joint replacement relieves pain and often improves movement, but complications are not uncommon and tend to increase with time after a replacement.

Infection (Fig. 16) will cause painful loosening and removal of the prosthesis is then necessary, resulting in an excision arthroplasty (Fig. 13).

Mechanical failure of the components can occur (Fig. 17).

In addition an artificial joint may *dislocate*, or *heterotopic ossification* can occur around the joint.

See also osteoarthritis of spine (p. 79), hand (p. 107), hip (p. 117), knee (p. 129) and foot (p. 147).

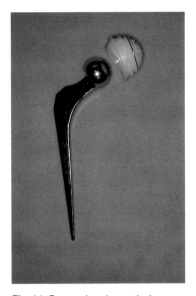

Fig. 14 Femoral and acetabular components of a total hip replacement.

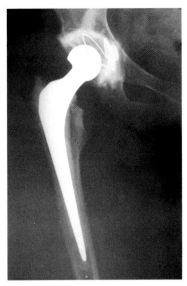

Fig. 15 Radiograph of a total hip replacement.

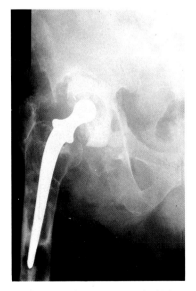

Fig. 16 An infected, loose, total hip replacement.

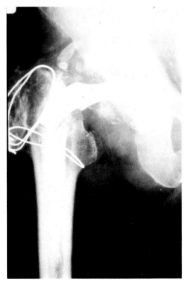

Fig. 17 Mechanical failure of the stem of a total hip replacement.

Arthritis (3)

Rheumatoid arthritis

A common (2–5% of adults in Britain) polyarthritis characterised by proliferation of the synovial lining of joints.

Cause

Unknown. An immunological basis seems likely.

Pathology

A chronic proliferative synovitis that causes stretching of joint capsules and ligaments, rupture of tendons and eventually destruction of articular cartilage.

Clinical features

Usual age of onset is 'prime of life' (20–60 yr). Women more often affected than men. The disease usually affects the small joints of the hands and feet first in a symmetrical fashion. Morning stiffness, pain and swelling are prominent features. Occasionally one large joint, usually the knee, is involved initially. On examination there is palpable synovial thickening in joints or around the tendons (Fig. 18). There may be joint effusions and warmth and erythema may be early features. Rheumatoid nodules are classically found on the extensor aspect of the forearm near the elbow (Fig. 19) but are not always present.

Investigations

Radiographs show periarticular osteoporosis. Erosions may be seen—small 'bites' from bones adjacent to joints, best seen in the metacarpo or metatarsophalangeal joints (Fig. 20). Loss of joint space, bone destruction and deformity are later features.

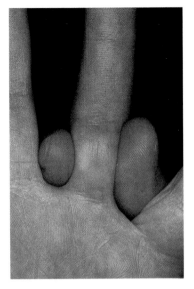

Fig. 18 Flexor synovitis in a finger.

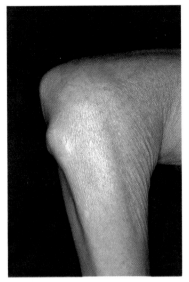

Fig. 19 A typical rheumatoid nodule.

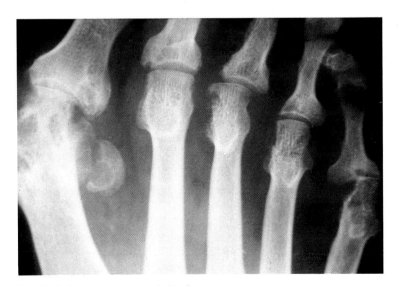

Fig. 20 Periarticular erosions in the foot.

Rheumatoid arthritis (contd)

Course

Initial episode may settle leaving little functional disability, but further attacks may occur. In most patients the disease is chronic with exacerbations, but may eventually 'burn out'. Progressive destruction of joints in the hands (Fig. 21), feet (Fig. 22) and the major weight bearing joints (Fig. 23) produces severe disability.

Treatment

Relief of pain by drugs and rest in splints.
Provision of appliances to help with the activities of daily living.
Social support, including help with appropriate employment.
Surgical treatment. Surgical treatment is indicated mainly in patients with severe disability and deformity.
A joint assessment by rheumatologist, orthopaedic surgeon, occupational therapist and physiotherapist is essential.
Operations are designed to relieve pain and increase function. The general types of procedure are:
Soft tissue repairs. For example, repair of ruptured tendons.
Synovectomy. Removal of synovial lining. Must be done before the articular cartilage is damaged.
Osteotomy (p. 7). Occasionally indicated if joint destruction is not advanced.
Arthrodesis (p. 7). Particularly for small joints in hand, wrist and ankle.
Arthroplasty (p. 9). Excision arthroplasty is used in the forefoot and replacement arthroplasty in the hip and knee.

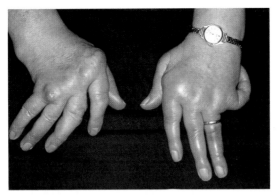

Fig. 21 Rheumatoid arthritis affecting the hands.

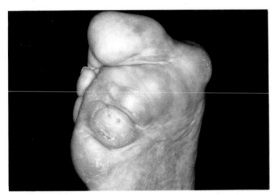

Fig. 22 Typical changes of severe rheumatoid arthritis in the forefoot.

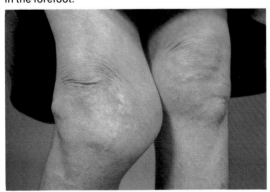

Fig. 23 A valgus deformity of the knee secondary to rheumatoid arthritis.

Ankylosing spondylitis

A chronic inflammatory disorder, typically affecting the spine and sacroiliac joints, which leads to ossification of ligaments. Fairly common (about 1 in 200 men, but less often affects women).

Clinical features

Onset in 18–30 age group.
Early. Low back pain which typically wakens the patient in the morning. Peripheral joints are affected in about 10%. Common clinical findings are limitation of spinal movements and chest expansion.
Late. Without treatment there is a tendency for the spine and other affected joints to become stiffer. Progressive kyphosis can occur, making it difficult for the patient to see ahead (Fig. 24).

Investigations

Radiographs of the spine classically show calcification of the intervertebral ligaments, eventually producing a 'bamboo spine' (Fig. 25), but such radiological appearances should be unusual with early vigorous treatment. The sacroiliac joints are usually narrow and sclerotic (Fig. 26).
ESR usually raised in early active phase. HLA B27 antigen is present in 95% of patients. (This is *not* a diagnostic test since many unaffected people have the same antigen.)

Treatment

Early. Active exercise programme to prevent stiffness. Anti-inflammatory analgesic drugs.
Late. Total hip replacement for stiff hips. Rarely, spinal osteotomy for severe deformity.

GENERAL ORTHOPAEDICS

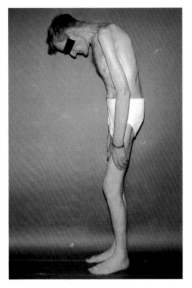

Fig. 24 Typical spinal deformity of severe ankylosing spondylitis.

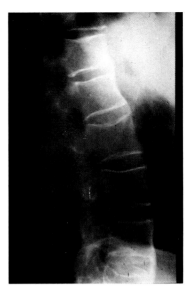

Fig. 25 'Bamboo spine' in ankylosing spondylitis.

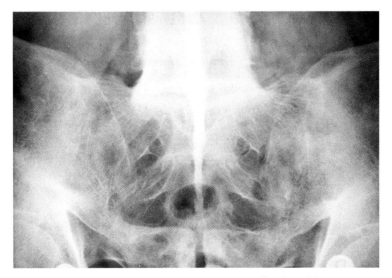

Fig. 26 Obliteration of the sacroiliac joints. Note ossification of the interspinous ligament.

Gout

A metabolic disorder characterised by hyperuricaemia and deposition of urate crystals. May be secondary to polycythaemia and myeloproliferative disorders, or precipitated by trauma (including surgery), dietary indiscretions or certain drugs, notably diuretics.

Clinical features

More common in men. Usually one joint (typically the metatarsophalangeal joint of the big toe) is affected, with acute onset of pain, redness and swelling.
Later there is a chronic arthritis with deposition of tophi and destruction of the joint (Figs 27, 28).

Treatment

An acute attack is treated with anti-inflammatory drugs and further attacks are prevented by long-term treatment with uricosuric agents. Surgical treatment is rarely necessary.

Chondrocalcinosis (pyrophosphate arthropathy; pseudogout)

Accumulation of crystals of calcium pyrophosphate within joints.

Clincial features

Like gout, it is commonest around 60 years, but the incidence is the same in men and women. One joint is affected, usually the knee. In the acute attack there is swelling, redness and pain, stiffness and effusions.
Radiographs show calcification of cartilage (Fig. 29). Fluid aspirated from the joint is turbid and laden with leucocytes. Under polarised light weakly birefringent crystals can be seen.

Treatment

Anti-inflammatory analgesics.

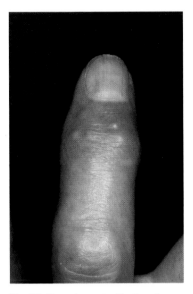

Fig. 27 Chronic gout affecting the distal interphalangeal joint.

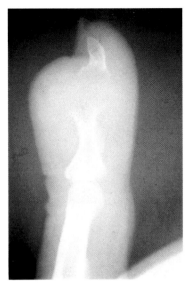

Fig. 28 Destruction of the distal interphalangeal joint due to gout.

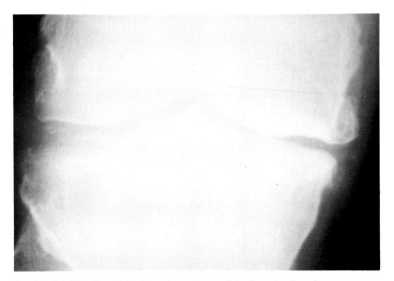

Fig. 29 Calcification of the lateral meniscus of the knee in chondro-calcinosis.

Arthritis (7)

Psoriatic arthropathy

Occurs in 10% of people with psoriasis.

Clinical features

Skin disorder may not be marked. Many patients who develop arthritis have only thickening (hyperkeratosis) or pitting of the nails (Fig. 30). Arthritis can affect any joint, but typically involves the small joints of the hands. Onset may be acute, with erythema and swelling. Later features are similar to rheumatoid arthritis with severe destructive arthropathy affecting the hands and feet.

Treatment

Analgesic and anti-inflammatory drugs. Surgical arthrodesis of small joints if pain and instability warrant it.

Alkaptonuria (ochronosis)

An uncommon disease, transmitted as an autosomal recessive trait, in which there is excessive excretion of homogentisic acid in the urine and deposition of black pigment in tissues.

Clinical features

Onset of back pain and stiffness in 20–40 age group. More common in men. Knees and shoulders often affected. Arthritis is chronic and progressive.
Radiographs show narrowing of disc spaces and sclerosis of the adjacent vertebral end plates (Fig. 31). Changes in other joints are similar to osteoarthritis.

Treatment

Analgesic drugs.

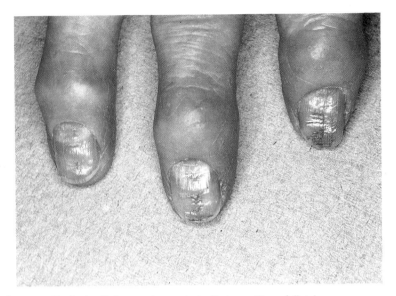

Fig. 30 Typical nail changes in psoriasis. Note swelling of distal interphalangeal joints.

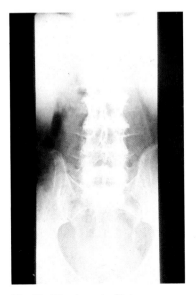

Fig. 31 Alkaptonuria. Note narrowing of disc spaces.

Haemophilic arthropathy

Haemophilia is a disorder of the blood-clotting mechanism due to deficiency of Factor VIII. It is transmitted as an X-linked recessive trait and therefore it is almost always males who are affected.

Clinical features

Recurrent haemarthroses (Fig. 32) cause painful swelling of joints and eventually produce a chronic arthropathy. The knees are most often involved but elbows, shoulders, wrists and hips may be affected. The joint involvement is usually asymmetrical. Radiographs are initially normal but later show loss of joint space and a characteristic squaring of the epiphysis (Fig. 33).

Treatment

Immobilisation, replacement of Factor VIII, analgesia, prevention of joint contractures by splinting.

Reiter's syndrome

A reactive arthritis may follow bacillary dysentery or sexually acquired non-specific urethritis.

Clinical features

More common in men and usually starts 2 – 3 weeks after infection. Arthritis may affect feet, ankles or knees and is asymmetrical, affecting one or a few joints. Conjunctivitis, skin lesions on the soles of the feet (keratoderma) (Fig. 34) and plantar fasciitis (p. 131) are common features.

Treatment

The urethral discharge is treated with tetracyclines. Arthritis is treated by rest, splintage and anti-inflammatory analgesics. Recurrent arthritis is quite common.

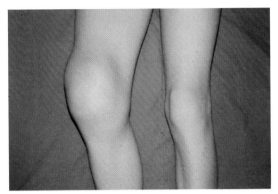

Fig. 32 Haemarthrosis in right knee due to haemophilia.

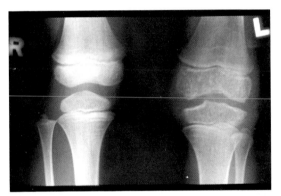

Fig. 33 Radiological changes in left knee due to haemophilia.

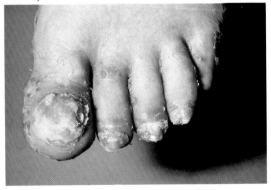

Fig. 34 Reiter's syndrome. Swollen toes and skin changes of keratoderma blenorrhagica.

3 | Neuromuscular Disorders (1)

Cerebral palsy

Non-progressive brain damage affecting upper motor neurone function and often resulting in poor control of voluntary muscles.

Causes

Cerebral maldevelopment, fetal anoxia, birth trauma, infections and head injuries.

Incidence

Around 2 per 1000 children of school age.

Classification

By limbs affected. e.g. hemiplegia, diplegia, quadriplegia (Fig. 35).
By pattern of muscle dysfunction. Spastic (increased tone), athetoid (uncontrolled writhing movements), ataxic (poor co-ordination), rigid or mixed.

Clinical features

Varies with type of cerebral palsy. Locomotor disability is only one aspect; there may be mental deficiency, although this is not invariable, and disorders of speech, vision and hearing are common.

Management

A team approach is important. The paediatrician, psychologist, physiotherapist and many other specialists will be involved in helping the child and family.

Orthopaedic aspects

Spasm of muscles causes limbs to be held in abnormal positions and fixed deformities may occur. Typical deformities are flexion of the elbow and wrist, adduction of hips, flexion of knees and plantar flexion (equinus) of foot (Fig. 36). Imbalance between spastic hip adductors and weak abductors may cause subluxation or even dislocation of hip (Fig. 37). Deformities can be minimised by muscle training, splinting and bracing. In carefully selected patients operations such as tendon elongation, tendon transfer, arthrodesis and muscle denervation may be used.

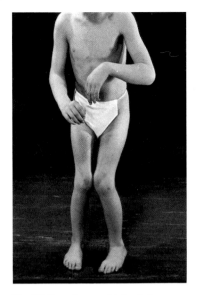

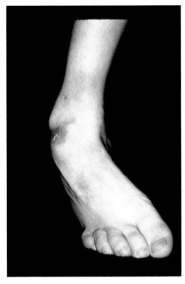

Fig. 35 Spastic quadriplegia in cerebral palsy.

Fig. 36 Equinus deformity of the foot in cerebral palsy.

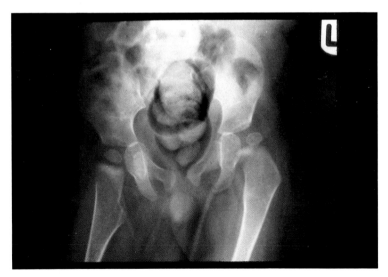

Fig. 37 Subluxation of the left hip in a child with cerebral palsy.

Poliomyelitis

An infectious disease usually affecting children, caused by one of the polioviruses, which have an affinity for the motor neurones of the anterior horn of the spinal cord and brain stem. Can occur as an epidemic in an unvaccinated population.

Clinical features

The disease is mild in most cases, causing no more than a flu-like illness with gastrointestinal upset.
If the anterior horn cells are damaged there is paralysis of the appropriate muscles.
Paralysis may be partial or complete, temporary or permanent, depending on the extent and severity of neurological involvement. The disease can be divided into five stages:
1. Incubation—14 days
2. Onset—2 days
3. Severe paralysis—approximately 2 months
4. Recovery of paralysis—up to 2 years
5. Residual paralysis—permanent.

Orthopaedic aspects

Total paralysis will render a limb flail. An appropriate orthosis for the leg will allow weight bearing.
Partial paralysis produces an imbalance in strength between groups of muscles and this can lead to deformity, particularly in the growing child (Figs 38, 39).
Mobile deformities can be minimised by splinting or tendon transfers to rebalance muscle actions.
Fixed deformities may require correction by osteotomy, or arthrodesis of joints.

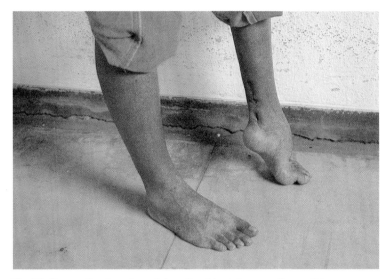

Fig. 38 Severe fixed equinus deformity of foot due to poliomyelitis.

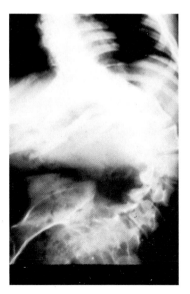

Fig. 39 A gross scoliosis attributable to imbalance of muscles acting on the spine.

Neuromuscular Disorders (3)

Muscular dystrophies

Disorders in which there are primary pathological changes within muscles, giving rise to progressive weakness. Three examples will be given, to illustrate some orthopaedic aspects of these conditions.

Pseudohypertrophic (Duchenne) muscular dystrophy. Transmitted as a sex-linked recessive characteristic, and therefore typically affects boys. Onset aged 3–5 with weakness and a tendency to fall; child 'climbs up his legs' to straighten up (Fig. 40) because of weakness in the hip extensors. Heel cords may become tight. Eventually the child is confined to a wheelchair and death from respiratory complications occurs towards the end of the second decade.

Congenital myopathies. Various types are recognised; typical features are 'floppiness' in babies and weakness in young children. Orthopaedic features include dislocation of the hips (p. 109), flat feet (p. 137) and scoliosis (Fig. 41). Supporting orthoses may allow the child to start walking, and surgical treatment of deformities, particularly scoliosis, is sometimes needed.

Facioscapulohumeral muscular dystrophy. Usually autosomal dominant transmission. Manifest in second decade with weakness and wasting of muscles around shoulders, mouth and eyes. Life expectation is good and stabilisation of the scapulae may improve function of the shoulders (Fig. 42).

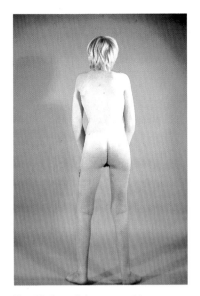

Fig. 40 Pseudohypertrophic muscular dystrophy.

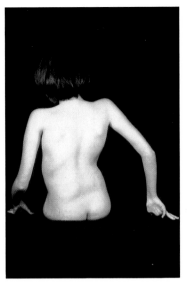

Fig. 41 Scoliosis due to weak trunk muscles in a congenital myopathy.

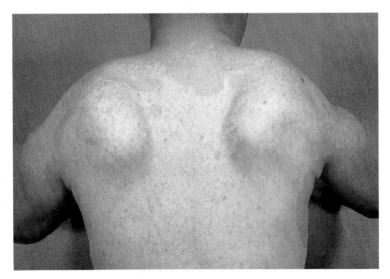

Fig. 42 Facioscapulohumeral dystrophy.

Neuromuscular Disorders (4)

Spina bifida

Failure of closure of the vertebral canal during embryological development, frequently associated with malformation of the spinal cord and nerve roots.

Clinical features

These depend on the severity of malformation of the nervous system. Tethering of nerve roots may cause only minor foot deformities but in severe forms (Fig. 43) there will be extensive paralysis and sensory loss in the lower limbs and loss of neurological control of pelvic viscera resulting in incontinence. Hydrocephalus is common in severe spina bifida because of blockage in the circulation of cerebrospinal fluid.

Orthopaedic aspects

Children with severe spina bifida who survive the neonatal period will often need correction of lower limb deformities and fitting of orthoses to allow walking. Gross spinal deformities can develop as the child grows.

Arthrogryphosis multiplex congenita

A rare congenital condition of unknown cause in which the limb muscles fail to develop.

Clinical features

Variable, depending on extent of the disorder. The involvement is usually symmetrical and the lower limbs are affected more than the upper. The limbs are thin. Joints are stiff and often dislocated. Club foot deformity is common (Fig. 44).

Treatment

Deformities are difficult or impossible to correct surgically. Function is often surprisingly good.

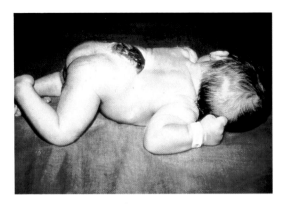

Fig. 43 Severe spina bifida.

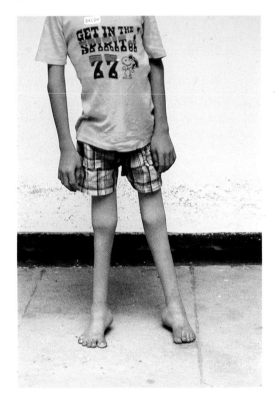

Fig. 44 Arthrogryphosis.

Peroneal muscular atrophy (Charcot-Marie-Tooth disease)

A not uncommon hereditary neuropathy, usually transmitted as an autosomal dominant trait.

Clinical features

Weakness and wasting of intrinsic muscles in the foot leading to pes cavus (Fig. 45) and clawing of toes which are usually manifest by 5–10 years. Weakness of calf muscles is common and the hands and forearms may be involved. Ankle jerk reflex is often lost and there is diminution of vibration sense below the knee.

Treatment

See treatment of pes cavus (p. 135).

Neuropathic arthropathy (Charcot's joints)

Disorganisation of a joint secondary to diminished pain sensation. Classically due to tabes dorsalis form of syphilis, but now more often caused by diabetes mellitus or occasionally syringomyelia.

Clinical features

Joint involved depends to some extent on underlying cause, the joints of the lower limbs being more often affected in tabes and diabetes and the upper limb joints in syringomyelia. Condition may start as acute swelling and discomfort; later there is progressive destruction with deformity and instability of the involved joint, but pain may be slight (Fig. 46).

Treatment

Early. Rest and analgesics.
Late. Stabilisation by an orthosis when there is destruction and instability. Surgical arthrodesis is notoriously difficult to achieve.

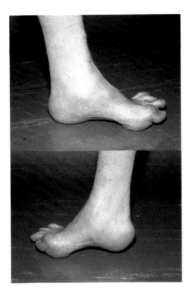

Fig. 45 Cavus foot in peroneal muscular atrophy.

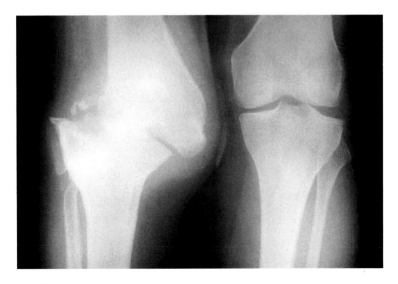

Fig. 46 Neuropathic destruction of the right knee.

Skeletal dysplasias (1)

A large group of congenital disorders which are characterised by generalised skeletal and often soft tissue abnormalities. Many, but not all, are heritable. Most are uncommon, and some are extremely rare. Some of the more common and important disorders will be illustrated.

Osteogenesis imperfecta (fragilitas ossium; 'brittle bone disease')

A group of disorders due to abnormal collagen synthesis, in which all bones in the skeleton are abnormally soft and break easily.

Clinical features

Two main subtypes:
Congenita. More severe form. Children may be born with fractures. Dwarfing and deformity often severe in survivors. Sporadic or autosomal recessive pattern of inheritance.
Tarda. More common form, Fractures become frequent in early childhood but their number becomes less as the child gets older. Autosomal dominant inheritance.
In both types there may be blue discoloration of the sclerae (Fig. 47), ligamentous laxity and poor wound healing.
X-ray examination shows slender bones (Fig. 48). Multiple fractures at different stages of healing may lead to confusion with a 'battered baby'. In severe cases repeated fractures lead to gross deformity of long bones (Fig. 49).

Treatment

Fractures usually heal with routine treatment. Severe bowing of long bones can be corrected by multiple osteotomies and stabilisation with intramedullary rods. Intramedullary rods are also used to prevent fractures.

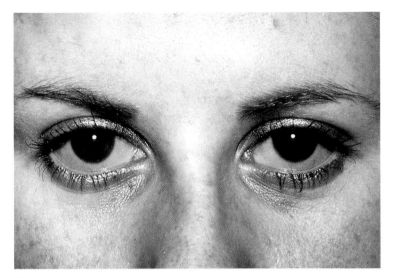

Fig. 47 Blue sclerae in osteogenesis imperfecta.

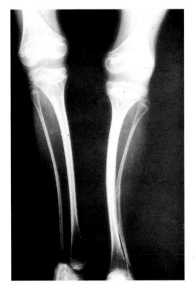

Fig. 48 Typical slender bones.

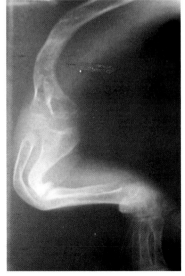

Fig. 49 Severe bowing due to repeated fractures.

Skeletal Dysplasias (2)

Achondroplasia

A relatively common disorder in which the limbs are short, but growth of the trunk is almost normal. Autosomal dominant inheritance.

Clinical features

Short limbs, short broad hands ('trident hands'), relative enlargement of the head, coarse facial features and lumbar lordosis (Fig. 50).

Treatment

Not usually needed, but the lumbar spinal canal is narrow in achondroplastic individuals and neurological complications due to spinal stenosis (p. 79) sometimes occur.

The mucopolysaccharidoses

A group of disorders characterised by abnormal storage of mucopolysaccharides due to absence of enzymes necessary for their metabolism. Like all congenital dosorders in which there is an enzyme deficiency there is a recessive pattern of inheritance.

Clinical features

Often not apparent at birth. Later mental deficiency, dwarfing, hepatosplenomegaly and various skeletal deformities may develop. The clinical picture varies with the particular type of enzyme deficiency.
A striking feature of Morquio's disease (mucopolysaccharidosis IV, in which there is inability to metabolise keratan sulphate) is the protruding sternum (Fig. 51). Dwarfing is marked and the hands are short (Fig. 52).

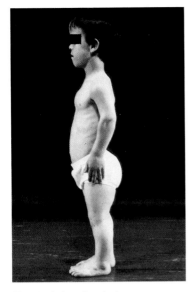

Fig. 50 Achondroplasia.

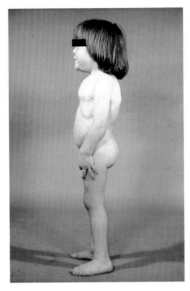

Fig. 51 Morquio's disease.

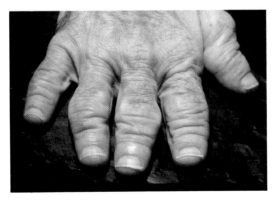

Fig. 52 The hand of a patient with Morquio's disease.

Diaphyseal aclasis (multiple exostoses)

A fairly common disorder, of autosomal dominant inheritance, in which exostoses form in the metaphyseal region of long bones.

Clinical features

Palpable bony lumps, typically around knees (Fig. 53), ankles and shoulders. The exostoses are bony outgrowths with cartilaginous caps and are therefore usually larger than they appear radiologically.

Extensive involvement may be associated with short stature and deformity of limbs. Very rarely malignant change can occur.

Treatment

Removal of unsightly exostoses or those causing pressure effects, e.g. on nerves.

See also osteochondroma (p. 49).

Ollier's disease (multiple enchondromatosis; dyschondroplasia)

A rare congenital disease, characterised by persistence of unmineralised cartilage within long bones. Sporadic in occurrence, with no genetic basis.

Clinical features

Usually asymmetrical involvement. Hands are frequently affected by multiple cartilaginous 'tumours' or hamartomas (Fig. 54) that are often large and unsightly (Fig. 55). Extensive lesions may cause shortening and deformities in limbs. Malignant change to a chondrosarcoma can occur.

Treatment

Corrective osteotomy of deformed bones, or amputation of severely involved, functionally useless parts.

See also enchondroma (p. 49) and chondrosarcoma (p. 55).

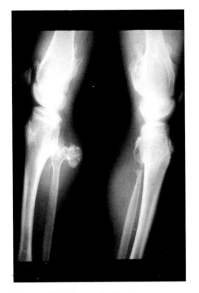

Fig. 53 Diaphyseal aclasis.

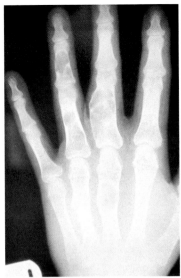

Fig. 54 Ollier's disease.

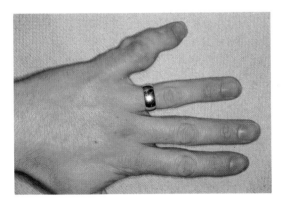

Fig. 55 Ollier's disease.

Multiple epiphyseal dysplasia

The epiphyses of many bones develop abnormally. There may be several types but one large group is certainly of autosomal dominant inheritance.

Clinical features

Clinically apparent during childhood. The epiphyses are small, mottled and irregular. Typically the epiphyses of long bones in the lower limbs are worst affected, and the appearance of the hips may be mistaken for bilateral Perthes' disease (p. 113). Short stature and mild deformities are common (Fig. 56). Hands and feet are often short and stubby. Osteoarthritis may occur at an early age, particularly affecting the hips (Fig. 57).

Treatment

Medical and surgical management of osteoarthritis (p. 7).

Osteopetrosis

Abnormal remodelling of bone causes osteosclerosis, obliteration of marrow cavities and brittleness of bones. The condition is due to abnormal function of osteoclasts. Severe (congenita) and mild (tarda) forms are recognised, the inheritance being autosomal recessive and dominant, respectively.

Clinical features

Congenita form is present at birth. In the tarda form fractures occur during childhood. Osteopetrosis congenita has a poor prognosis and the infant often develops a severe anaemia due to obliteration of the marrow cavities. Radiographs show dense bones with abnormal modelling (Fig. 58).

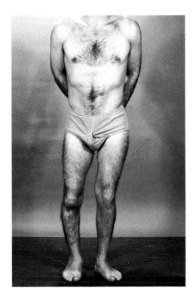

Fig. 56 Deformity in multiple epiphyseal dysplasia.

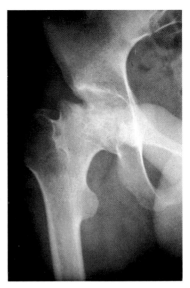

Fig. 57 Osteoarthritis of the hip in multiple epiphyseal dysplasia.

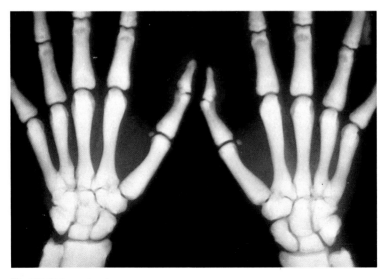

Fig. 58 Osteopetrosis.

Fibrous dysplasia

Replacement of parts of bones by fibrous tissue. The cause is unknown and there is no hereditary element.

One bone or several may be involved (monostotic and polyostotic forms). Usually the lesions are found in the shafts and metaphyses of long bones.

Clinical features

The lesions may be asymtomatic, or may present as local enlargement or deformity of the affected bone or bones (Fig. 59). Pathological fractures can occur and gross deformities can be produced if the disease is progressive. Polyostotic fibrous dysplasia is sometimes accompanied by extensive skin pigmentation (Albright's syndrome, Fig. 60).

Investigations

Radiographs show expansion of the bone, with thinning of the cortex. The abnormal area may have a 'ground glass' appearance. Similar appearances are found in hyperparathyroidism, which may be distinguished from fibrous dysplasia by biochemical evidence of abnormal calcium homeostasis.

In severe cases there will be radiological evidence of pathological fractures and deformities (Fig. 61).

Treatment

Fractures are treated by standard methods. Corrective osteotomy of deformed bone may be necessary.

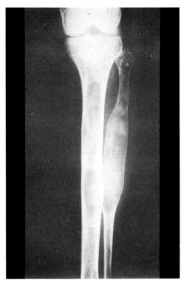

Fig. 59 Fibrous dysplasia affecting the tibia and fibula.

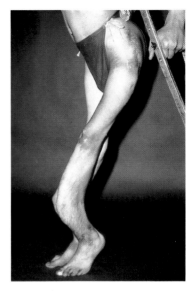

Fig. 60 Albright's syndrome.

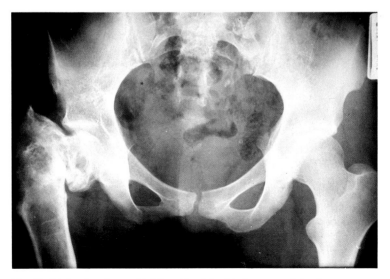

Fig. 61 A 'shepherd's crook' deformity of the hip (coxa vara) due to fibrous dysplasia.

| # Skeletal Dysplasias (6)

Neurofibromatosis (von Recklinghausen's disease)

A condition in which there is skin pigmentation, tumours within peripheral nerves, overgrowth of tissue and sometimes skeletal deformities. Autosomal dominant inheritance.

Clinical features

The manifestations of this condition are variable in extent and severity. 'Café au lait' skin patches (Fig. 62) and cutaneous fibromata and neurofibromata (Fig. 63) are the typical findings. Neurofibromata forming on peripheral nerves within the vertebral canal can compress the spinal cord. Malignant change may occur in neurofibromata. In severely affected individuals there may be local gigantism and a gross scoliosis (p. 71) can develop.

Congenital pseudarthrosis of the tibia (Fig. 64) is a curious condition that is associated with neurofibromatosis. During early childhood the tibia becomes progressively deformed.

Treatment

Large, unsightly neurofibromata, or those causing local pressure effects, should be excised. Early spinal fusion is usually necessary for an increasing scoliosis.

Congenital pseudarthrosis of the tibia is notoriously difficult to treat; repeated bone grafting procedures often fail to secure union.

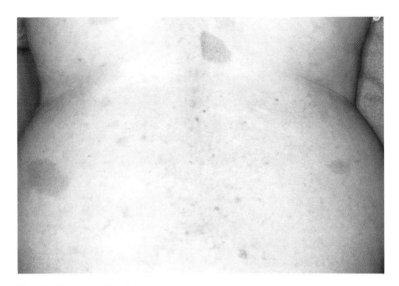

Fig. 62 'Café au lait' patches.

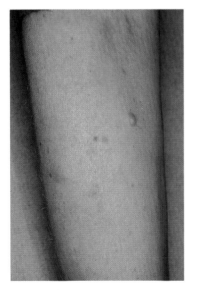

Fig. 63 Cutaneous neurofibromata.

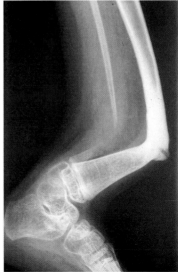

Fig. 64 Pseudarthrosis of the tibia.

4 | Skeletal Dysplasias (7)

Marfan's syndrome (arachnodactyly)

An uncommon condition characterised by abnormal height and long thin extremities. Autosomal dominant inheritance.

Clinical features

Manifestations are variable but the individual is usually tall with long slender fingers (Fig. 65) and toes. Generalised laxity of connective tissue may cause dislocation of the lenses of the eyes, aortic dilatation and incompetence. High arched palate and prognathism are common.

Orthopaedic aspects

Because of joint laxity patients are prone to develop flat feet (p. 137), genu recurvatum, recurrent dislocation of the patellae (p. 125) and spinal deformities, notably kyphosis and scoliosis (p. 71).

Ehlers–Danlos syndrome

A syndrome characterised by joint and skin laxity and a haemorrhagic tendency. Mild forms are probably quite common but severe involvement (as seen in the 'indiarubber men' of side shows) is rare. Autosomal dominant inheritance.

Clinical features

Joints are hyperextensible (Fig. 66). Recurrent dislocations of hips, patellae and shoulders are liable to occur. Scoliosis, kyphosis and foot deformities are not uncommon. The skin is lax and is prone to heal poorly with 'tissue paper' scars especially over the knees (Fig. 67) and elbows.

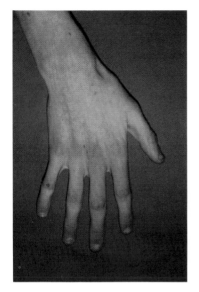

Fig. 65 The hand in Marfan's syndrome.

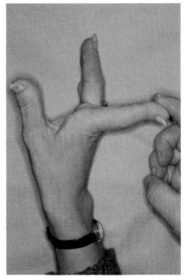

Fig. 66 Hyperextensible joints in the Ehlers–Danlos syndrome.

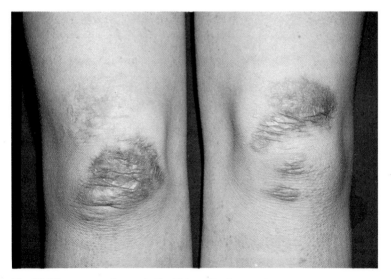

Fig. 67 'Tissue paper' scars in the Ehlers–Danlos syndrome.

5 | Local Disorders of Bone

Fibrous cortical defect

A common lesion which is usually an incidental x-ray finding in children aged 10–15. Cause unknown.
Radiographic appearance is characteristic. The lesion is eccentrically placed, initially in the metaphyseal region, but later moving away from the epiphyseal growth plate. Overlying cortex is thin or absent. Femur is most commonly involved (Fig. 68).

Treatment

Not needed. Disappears in 2–5 years.

Solitary bone cyst (unicameral bone cyst)

May present during childhood as a pathological fracture. More common in boys. Usually found in proximal part of humerus (Fig. 69) or femur.

Treatment

Fractures usually heal, but may recur. The cyst often disappears spontaneously and obliteration has been shown to be hastened by injection of methylprednisolone acetate into the cyst.

Bone infarct/avascular necrosis

Loss of blood supply causes local death of bone. The condition is often idiopathic but may be seen in divers or tunnel workers ('caisson disease'), in association with alcoholism or steroid treatment, or after trauma.

Clinical features

An infarct in the diaphysis of a long bone (Fig. 70) is often asymptomatic. However, when bone adjacent to a joint is involved there may be loss of support of articular cartilage, and secondary osteoarthritis is common.

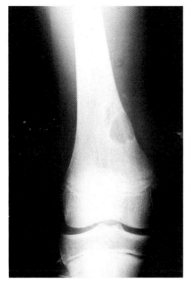

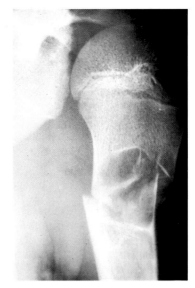

Fig. 68 Fibrous cortical defect.

Fig. 69 Fracture through a solitary bone cyst.

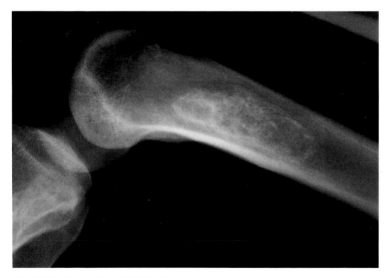

Fig. 70 Medullary infarct in the femur.

Bone Tumours (1)

Diagnosis

Depends on careful assessment of clinical, radiological and pathological features. Atypical radiological appearances are common.

Osteochondroma

Commonest benign bone tumour, often found near the knee (Fig. 71). Probably arises from the growth plate and consists of a bony spur covered by a large cap of cartilage which is radiolucent and therefore not seen on radiographs. If large and troublesome the lesion should be removed. See also diaphlyseal aclasis (p. 37).

Chondroma

A benign cartilaginous tumour arising within bone (enchondroma) or growing from it (ecchondroma). Common in hands (Fig. 72) and often presents as a pathological fracture. Healing is usually uneventful but curettage and bone grafting may be necessary.
See also multiple enchondromatosis (p. 37).

Osteoid Osteoma

A small vascular tumour consisting of osteoid tissue within a nidus of sclerotic bone. Usually found in children and young adults; common sites are small bones of hands and feet, neck of femur, tibia and spine. Causes pain which is typically worse at night and relieved specifically by aspirin. Sclerotic bone may be seen on radiographs, particularly tomographs, but they are often unremarkable; on an isotope bone scan the lesion is readily seen (Fig. 73). Treatment is by complete excision.

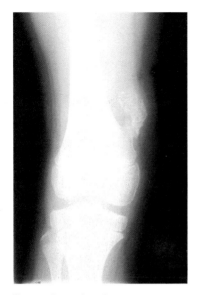

Fig. 71 Osteochondroma.

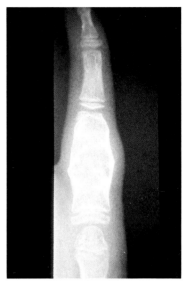

Fig. 72 Enchondroma in the proximal phalanx.

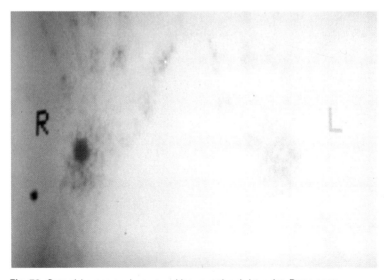

Fig. 73 Osteoid osteoma in a carpal bone at the right wrist. Bone scan.

Aneurysmal bone cyst

An expanded, blood-filled lesion typically found at the end of a long bone or the pedicle of a vertebra. May be caused by altered haemodynamics in bone rather than being a true neoplasm.

Clinical features

Most common in second and third decades of life. Produces pain, swelling (sometimes pulsatile) on bone, sometimes pathological fracture. Radiographs show a cystic lesion in the metaphyseal region of a long bone, not encroaching on the epiphysis (Fig. 74). Sometimes the cyst may 'explode' with loss of the overlying cortex.

Treatment

Drainage of the cyst and/or packing with bone chips. Radiotherapy is sometimes used if the lesion is surgically inaccessible.

Giant cell tumour (osteoclastoma)

Giant cells may be apparent histologically in these tumours, but their origin is not certain.

Clinical features

Usually occur in young adults. Common sites are lower end of radius, lower end of femur and upper end of tibia. The lesion causes pain and swelling; pathological fractures can occur. Radiographs show an expanded localised lesion in the metaphysis, extending up to the joint surface (Fig. 75).

Treatment

Excision if possible. Incomplete removal is a cause of local recurrence; rarely there is metastatic spread.

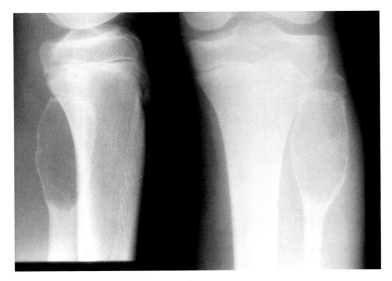

Fig. 74 Aneurysmal bone cyst in the fibula.

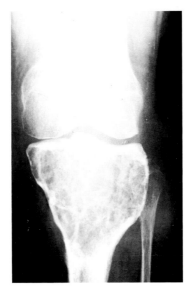

Fig. 75 Giant cell tumour in the tibia.

Osteosarcoma (osteogenic sarcoma)

A highly malignant tumour of bone-forming cells. Various histological subtypes are recognised.

Clinical features

Usually a tumour of children and young adults but it may be a complication of Paget's disease of bone (p. 65). Common sites (in young people) are the metaphyses of the upper end of the tibia, lower end of femur and upper end of humerus. The tumour causes pain, which may be worse at night, and swelling (Fig. 76). Pathological fractures can occur.

Radiographs show destruction of cortical bone and sometimes new bone formation beneath raised periosteum (Codman's triangle, Figs 77, 78). Isotope bone scan shows increased uptake at the site of the lesion. A CAT scan may show local soft tissue extension.

A biopsy, as in all bone tumours, is necessary for histological appraisal.

Treatment

Amputation well proximal to the tumour plus adjuvant chemotherapy. Local resection and reconstruction using custom-built prostheses may be possible for some tumours. Early metastasis to the lungs is common but survival has been improved by adjuvant chemotherapy. The parosteal variety of osteosarcoma (Fig. 79) has a relatively good prognosis after adequate resection but the prognosis for Paget's sarcoma is extremely poor.

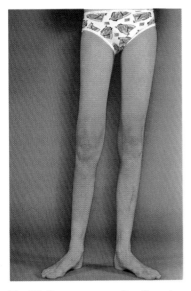

Fig. 76 Osteosarcoma. Swelling at the distal end of the right femur.

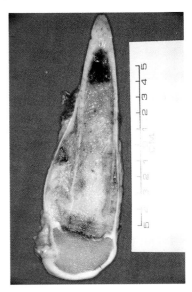

Fig. 77 Elevation of the periosteum by an osteosarcoma.

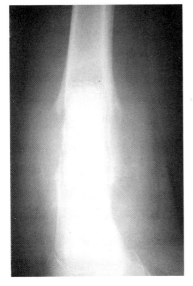

Fig. 78 Radiographic appearance of Codman's triangle.

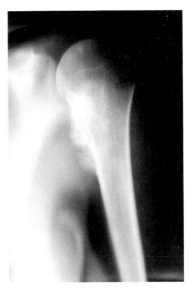

Fig. 79 A parosteal sarcoma of the humerus, shown by tomography.

| # Bone Tumours (4)

Chondrosarcoma

A malignant tumour derived from cartilage cells. Occasionally arises from pre-existing enchondromata or osteochondromata, especially when multiple (p. 37).

Clinical features

Usually occur in middle-aged people. There is a slowly-growing, painful lesion that may become very large (Fig. 80). Radiographs show either an expanding central lesion or a soft tissue shadow arising from the cortex of the bone. Areas of calcification within the tumour are characteristic (Fig. 81).

Treatment

Because of slow growth and late metastasis there is a relatively good prognosis after amputation well proximal to the tumour.

Ewing's tumour

A sarcomatous tumour of bone marrow. It may arise from endothelial cells or be a form of neuroblastoma.

Clinical features

Children are most often affected. Typically the tumour arises in the shaft of the tibia, femur or humerus, or in the pelvis (Fig. 82). There is local pain, swelling and warmth and often an intermittent pyrexia. Radiographs may show an 'onion skin' appearance due to deposition of successive layers of subperiosteal bone. The periosteal reaction may cause confusion with osteomyelitis, particularly as the ESR is often raised and there is a pyrexia.

Treatment

Amputation or radical radiotherapy often control the tumour for a time but the ultimate prognosis is usually poor since there is early metastatic spread to the lungs. Adjuvant chemotherapy may prolong survival.

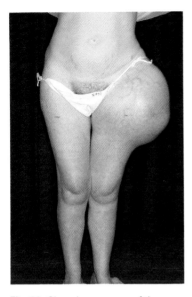 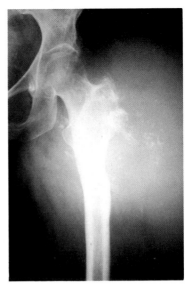

Fig. 80 Chondrosarcoma of the proximal part of the femur. A common site.

Fig. 81 Radiographic appearance showing calcification within the tumor.

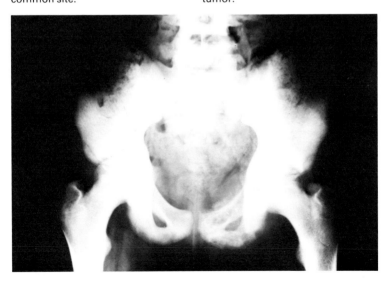

Fig. 82 Ewing's tumour affecting pubic rami on the left.

Multiple myeloma (plasmacytoma; myelomatosis)

Malignant tumour of plasma cells in marrow. May initially be solitary but has usually progressed to multiple stage on presentation. Vertebrae, ribs, skull and pelvis are common sites.

Clinical features

Bone pain, weakness, anaemia and weight loss. Investigations may show raised ESR, hypercalcaemia, abnormal proteins in serum and urine. Radiographs typically show vertebral collapse and sometimes 'pepper pot' lesions in the skull (Fig. 83).

Treatment

Chemotherapy, radiotherapy to local lesions. Prognosis is poor.

Metastatic bone tumours

Very common. Much more frequent than primary bone tumours. Typical primary tumours are situated in lung, breast, kidney and thyroid.

Clinical features

Pain, swelling, pathological fractures (Fig. 84).

Treatment

Isolated metastatic deposits warrant treatment to make the patient as comfortable as possible, even if the prognosis is poor. If technically possible internal stabilisation of bones should be carried out to prevent impending fractures from becoming complete. Internal fixation of complete fractures (Fig. 85) will relieve pain and minimise functional disability. Local treatment with radiotherapy may also be given. Pathological fractures often heal well.

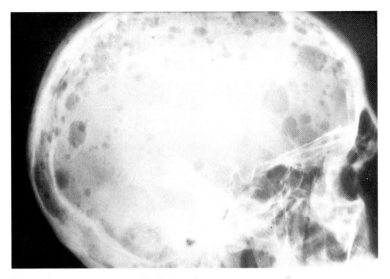

Fig. 83 Multiple myeloma. Skull deposits.

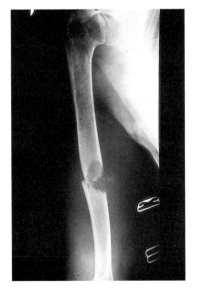

Fig. 84 Pathological fracture of the humerus due to metastatic tumour.

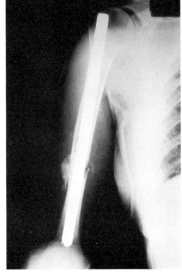

Fig. 85 Internal fixation for pathological fracture.

Synovial tumours

Synovial chondromatosis

An uncommon condition in which multiple cartilaginous foci form within synovial membranes. The cartilaginous foci may become calcified and often become detached resulting in loose bodies that can cause mechanical derangements of the affected joint.

Clinical features

30+ age group affected. Usually one joint is involved, the knee most frequently (Fig. 86). The joint swells and locks unpredictably when a loose body is trapped between the joint surfaces.

Treatment

Removal of loose bodies ± synovectomy.

Synoviosarcoma

A rare malignant mesothelial tumour.

Clinical features

Affects young adults. Presents as a slowly growing, often painful soft tissue swelling in the region of a joint, especially the joints of the lower limb.
Radiological examination reveals a soft tissue mass, sometimes with calcific stippling (Fig. 87).

Treatment

Local excision is inadequate and the tumour invariably recurs. Radical amputation is often necessary as the tumour is resistant to radio and chemotherapy. Metastasis to the lungs is common.

See also ganglion and villonodular synovitis (p. 97).

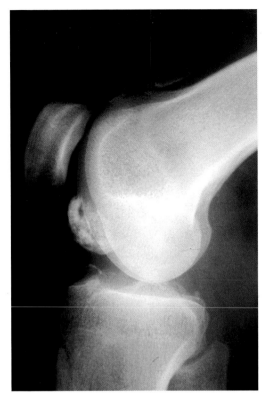

Fig. 86 Synovial chondromatosis.

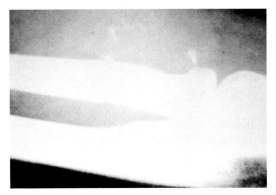

Fig. 87 Calcification within a synoviosarcoma.

| # Metabolic Bone Disease (1)

Osteoporosis

A generalised reduction in bone mass below the normal range for the particular age, sex and race of the individual. The bone is normal in quality but there is less of it than there should be.

Causes

Hormonal. Some bone loss is normal in the post-menopausal female, but if excessive can lead to clinically apparent osteoporosis. Also occurs in thyrotoxicosis and Cushing's syndrome.
Disuse. Immobilisation, weightlessness in astronauts.
Others. Rheumatoid arthritis (p. 11), osteogenesis imperfecta (p. 33), Marfan's syndrome (p. 45).

Clinical features

Often asymptomatic, but fractures through weak bone are very common. Usual sites are wrist (Colles' fracture), neck of humerus, vertebrae and neck of femur (Fig. 88). Back pain and loss of height are due to multiple vertebral compression fractures (Fig. 89) which may cause a dorsal kyphosis ('widow's hump', Fig. 90).

Investigations

Blood chemistry usually normal. Osteoporosis is not radiologically apparent until more than 30% of the total bone mass has been lost.

Treatment

Medical. There is no form of treatment that will reliably restore bone volume.
Surgical. Treatment of patients with fractures due to osteoporosis accounts for a major part of the workload of most orthopaedic surgeons.

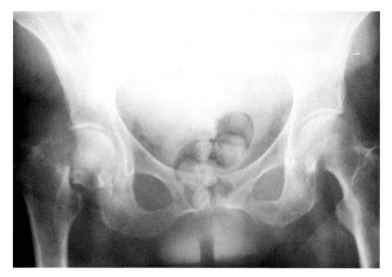

Fig. 88 A subcapital fracture of the right hip.

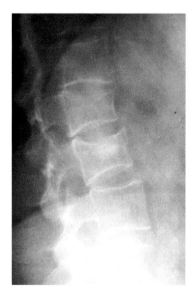

Fig. 89 Multiple vertebral fractures due to osteoporosis.

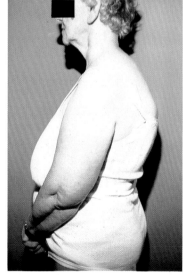

Fig. 90 Moderate kyphosis due to osteoporosis.

8 | Metabolic Bone Disease (2)

Osteomalacia and rickets are both due to inadequate intake or metabolism of vitamin D. Hypovitaminosis D results in poor mineralisation of the skeletal matrix. It may be nutritional or due to malabsorption or renal causes.

Rickets

The condition caused by hypovitaminosis D in childhood when bone growth is taking place.

Clinical features

Failure of mineralisation of the rapidly growing metaphyseal region of bones (Fig. 91) leads to swelling of bone ends and deformities (Fig. 92). There may be a waddling gait due to a proximal myopathy.

Investigations

Low serum calcium and phosphate, raised alkaline phosphatase. Typical X-ray features (Fig. 91).

Treatment

Adequate replacement and maintenance dosage of vitamin D. Deformities of long bones may not correct and osteotomy may be necessary.

Osteomalacia

The adult counterpart of rickets, usually affecting elderly people with poor diet.

Clinical features

Often unremarkable, but may present with generalised skeletal pain, weakness and fractures through weakened bone.

Investigations

Blood picture similar to rickets. Radiographs may show pseudofractures (Looser's zones) in the pubi rami (Fig. 93) and other bones.

Treatment

Adequate replacement and maintenance dosage of Vitamin D.
Treatment of fractures.

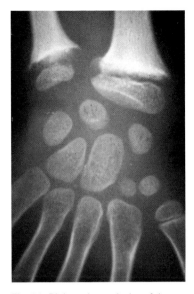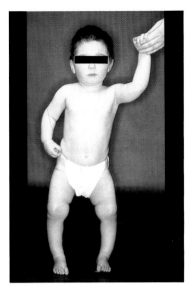

Fig. 91 Rickets. Irregularity of the metaphyses of the radius and ulna.

Fig. 92 Genu varum caused by rickets.

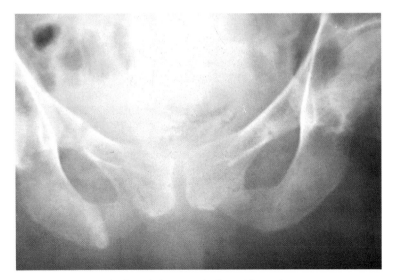

Fig. 93 Osteomalacia. Pseudofractures in the pubic rami.

Metabolic Bone Disease (3)

Paget's disease of bone (osteitis deformans)

Although loosely classified as a metabolic bone disease, Paget's disease of bone is a disorder of unknown aetiology in which there is thickening and deformity of one or several bones. The rates of deposition and resorption of bone appear to be out of phase.

Clinical features

Affects men more often than women. Becomes increasingly common with age, but rare below the age of 40.
Pelvis, femur, tibia, skull and vertebrae are common sites. Disease is asymptomatic in the majority, but it may cause pain, swelling and warmth over affected bones, which can become thickened and bowed (Fig. 94). Thickening of calvarium results in increase in head size and change of shape (Fig. 95).

Investigations

Plasma alkaline phosphatase raised, urinary hydroxyproline excretion increased. Localised osteoporosis is an early radiographic feature, but later there is coarse trabeculation, and loss of distinction between the cortex and medulla. Microfractures occur on the convex border of bones (Fig. 96).

Complications

Microfractures may progress to complete fractures (Fig. 97). Compression of nerves may cause deafness, or paraplegia. Osteoarthritis can occur when bone adjacent to a joint is affected. Osteosarcomatous change is uncommon; the prognosis is extremely poor.

Treatment

Medical. Analgesics, calcitonin, diphosphonates.
Surgical. Internal fixation of fractures is sometimes necessary.

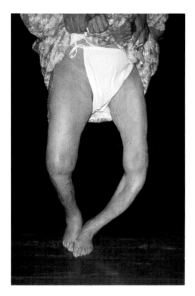

Fig. 94 Paget's disease affecting both legs.

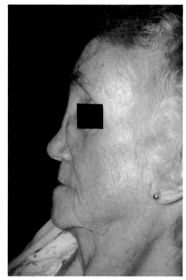

Fig. 95 Facial and skull changes in Paget's disease.

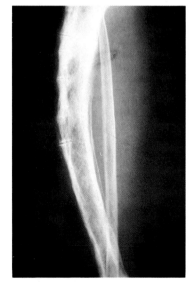

Fig. 96 Typical microfractures in the tibia.

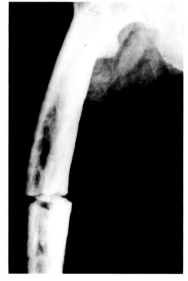

Fig. 97 A complete fracture of the femur.

Metabolic Bone Disease (4)

Vitamin C deficiency

Vitamin C is necessary for the formation of osteoid tissue. Severe lack of vitamin C is a rare cause of osteoporosis (p. 61).
In addition there is increased capillary fragility and in children minor injuries to bone may cause large subperiosteal haematomata, since the periosteum is only loosely attached to bone (Fig. 98). Secondary calcification of subperiosteal haematomata is followed by bony remodelling.

Fluorosis

Deposition of fluorine within the skeleton as fluorhydroxyapatite. Occurs in parts of the world where the drinking water has a high fluoride content (many times greater than the therapeutic levels used to prevent dental caries).
Bones are thick, sclerotic (Fig. 99) but brittle and therefore prone to fracture. Narrowing of the vertebral canal may cause spinal stenosis (p. 79).

Heavy metal poisoning

Ingested lead and other heavy metals may be deposited in the metaphyseal regions of growing bones (Fig. 100).
Other manifestations of lead poisoning such as gastrointestinal disorders and central nervous system symptoms are invariably present when the skeleton is affected.

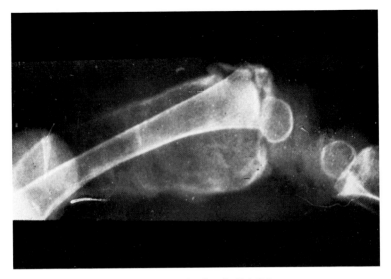

Fig. 98 Subperiosteal haemorrhage in vitamin C deficiency

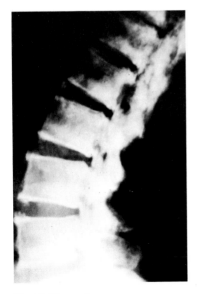

Fig. 99 Fluorosis.

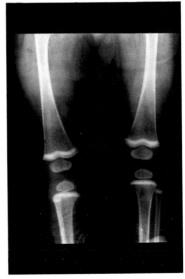

Fig. 100 Lead poisoning.

Torticollis

Tilting and rotation of the head.

Types

Infantile. Due to idiopathic contracture of one of the sternomastoid muscles (Fig. 101). Usually develops during infancy. Treatment is by stretching of the muscle or surgical division.
Secondary. Secondary to imbalance of extrinsic eye muscles, cervical lymphadenopathy or acute muscle spasm.
Spasmodic. A type of 'tic' in which there is sudden uncontrollable writhing of the neck. Cause unknown and no form of treatment has been found to be effective.

Cervical rib

An abnormal bony or fibrous development of the costal process of the 7th cervical vertebra (Fig. 102).

Clinical features

Often none, but vascular and neurological symptoms may occur and are attributed to pressure on the subclavian artery or lower trunks of the brachial plexus by the rib or a band attached to it. Young adults are usually affected.

Treatment

Mild symptoms respond to physiotherapy. Surgery is indicated only if there are objective, worsening neurological or vascular signs.

Congenital short neck (Klippel–Feil syndrome)

Shortening of the neck and limitation of movements due to multiple congenital anomalies of the cervical vertebrae. Sometimes there is webbing of the skin of the neck which can be improved surgically, but active treatment is seldom needed.

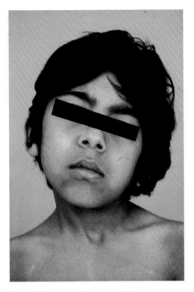

Fig. 101 Infantile torticollis.

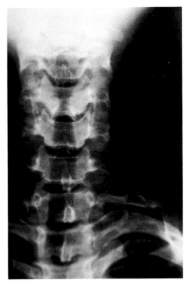

Fig. 102 Left cervical rib.

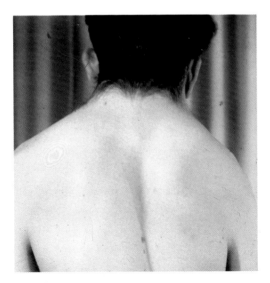

Fig. 103 Congenital short neck.

Scoliosis

Lateral curvature of the spine.

Classification

Postural. For example, a compensatory scoliosis occurs when one leg is shorter than the other. The spine is normal.

Structural. The curve is due to an abnormality of the spine. The two types can be distinguished by asking the patient to lean forwards (Fig. 104) when a postural scoliosis will disappear. Most structural curves are idiopathic in origin, but some are due to neuromuscular dysfunction (e.g. in poliomyelitis, muscular dystrophies) or congenital bony abnormalities in the spine (Fig. 105). Scoliosis is also a feature of many skeletal disorders (e.g. Marfan's syndrome, neurofibromatosis).

Clinical features

Depending on the cause the curve may commence at any age in a growing child. Any part of the thoracolumbar spine can be involved. Radiographs confirm the extent of the deformity (Fig. 106).

Treatment

Structural scoliosis gets worse during growth in most cases. Young children must be treated in a brace (the Milwaukee brace, or a modification) to prevent increasing deformity. In addition to the deformity, an untreated patient may have cardiorespiratory problems if the thoracic spine is involved. Older children are usually treated by surgical fusion of the affected spinal segment; often it is possible to correct residual deformity using implants (Harrington or Luque rods) that are attached to posterior elements of the vertebrae.

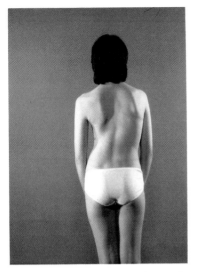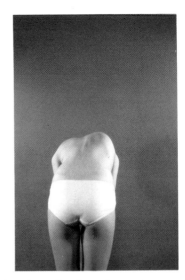

Fig. 104 A structural scoliosis remains when the patient leans forward.

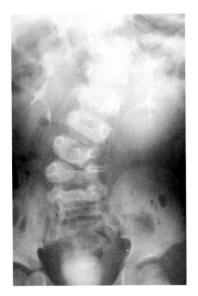

Fig. 105 Congenital vertebral abnormalities.

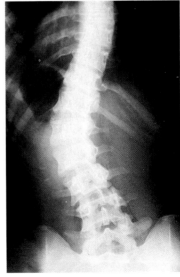

Fig. 106 A typical idiopathic scoliosis.

9 | Spine (3)

Discitis

An uncommon condition of unknown cause in which there is narrowing and sometimes calcification of the intervertebral disc space.

Clinical features

Affects children aged 6 – 14. The lumbar spine is usually involved. Child complains of pain in back or abdomen and is often pyrexial. Examination reveals muscle spasm and limitation of spinal movements. Radiological narrowing of the disc space (Fig. 107) may take a week or two to appear.

Treatment

Bed rest until symptoms settle.

Vertebra plana (Calvé's disease)

Collapse of a vertebral body, believed to be due to an eosinophilic granuloma of bone. Uncommon.

Clinical features

Affects children aged 2 – 10. There is local discomfort, usually in the thoracic spine. X-ray examination shows collapse of a vertebral body with preservation of disc spaces (Fig. 108).

Treatment

Rest until pain settles. The vertebral body may redevelop.

Adolescent kyphosis (Scheuermann's disease)

A common condition in which there is abnormal development of the ring epiphyses of the thoracic vertebral bodies.

Clinical features

Youngsters in the 12 – 16 age group develop a mild round-shouldered deformity (Fig. 109), sometimes associated with slight discomfort. Radiographs show wedging of vertebral bodies (Fig. 110).

Treatment

Seldom needed but in more severe cases a spinal brace may be used to prevent progression of the kyphosis.

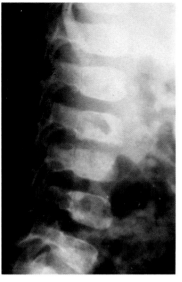

Fig. 107 Irregular disc space in discitis.

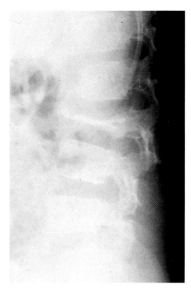

Fig. 108 Vertebra plana.

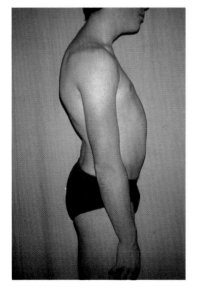

Fig. 109 Adolescent kyphosis.

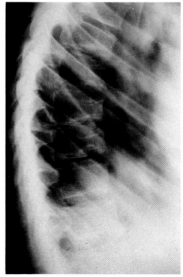

Fig. 110 Wedging of vertebra in adolescent kyphosis.

Spondylolisthesis

A defect in the pars interarticularis of a vertebra, usually occurring in the lower lumbar region, is known as a *spondylolysis* (Fig. 111). When it is associated with a forward slipping of one vertebra relative to another, or the sacrum, the condition is called a *spondylolisthesis* (Fig. 113).

Clinical features

Spondylolysis. May predispose adults to low back pain, but is also found incidentally in many adults who never suffer back pain.
Spondylolisthesis. Often due to a congenital or developmental abnormality of the vertebra and can cause low back pain in childhood. A step between the spinous processes may be palpable. Occasionally a sudden slip occurs and the youngster presents with a stiff spine, increased lumbar lordosis and hamstring spasm, causing the knees to be held in slight flexion (Fig. 112). Spondylolisthesis in adults is usually due to degenerative changes in the interfacetal joints of the vertebrae, but may be caused by injury or pathological fractures.

Treatment

Surgical fusion of the appropriate spinal segments is usually indicated for symptomatic spondylolisthesis in young people. In adults surgical treatment is seldom necessary and symptoms are relieved by wearing a spinal support.

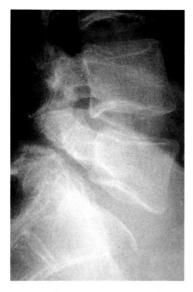

Fig. 111 Spondylolysis with defect in pars interarticularis of L5.

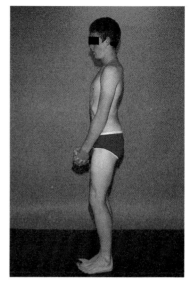

Fig. 112 Acute spondylolisthesis: the typical posture.

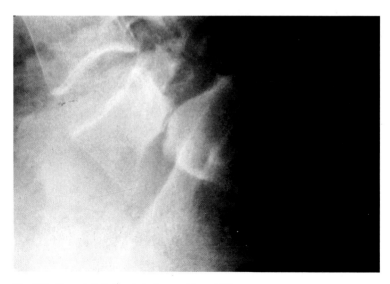

Fig. 113 Spondylolisthesis between L5 and S1.

Prolapsed intervertebral disc (slipped disc)

The gelatinous nucleus pulposus of an intervertebral disc may rupture through the annulus fibrosus, usually in a posterolateral direction, causing pressure on a nerve root. This often happens spontaneously but may follow acute strain while lifting.

Clinical features

Pressure on L5 or S1 nerve roots causes pain down the back of the leg (sciatica), often made worse by coughing. Normal lumbar lordosis is lost (Fig. 114) and spinal movements are restricted. To relieve pressure on the nerve the spine is held tilted to one side (Fig. 115); the direction of the tilt depends on the position of the prolapse in relation to the nerve root. Passive flexion of the hip with the knee held straight is limited (straight leg raising test) and pressing on the tibial nerve in the popliteal fossa causes pain. There may be motor and sensory impairment and loss of tendon jerks; the pattern will depend on the nerve root involved. Rarely a central disc prolapse will cause pressure on the cauda equina and urinary symptoms; this is a surgical emergency. Lumbar myelography or radiculography will show indentation of the dura at the level of the disc prolapse (Fig. 116).

Treatment

Most will settle with bed rest, analgesia and spinal support.
Surgical removal of the disc is considered only if sciatica or neurological signs fail to resolve with adequate conservative treatment, or if there is a central disc prolapse with cauda equina symptoms.

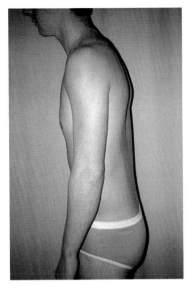

Fig. 114 Loss of lumbar lordosis in disc prolapse.

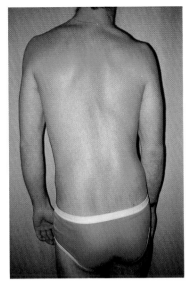

Fig. 115 Muscle spasm and lumbar spinal tilt.

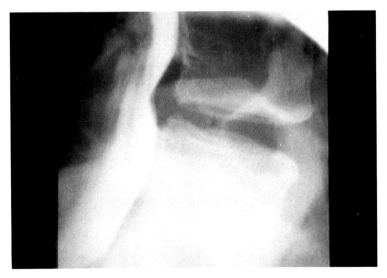

Fig. 116 Contrast radiograph showing disc prolapse at L5/S1 level.

9 | Spine (6)

Osteoarthritis

For a general description of osteoarthritis, see p. 7. Degenerative OA in the spine is extremely common. The clinical symptoms often bear little relationship to the severity of radiological changes. There are several clinical forms:

1. *Cervical spondylosis* (Fig. 117). Pain in the neck and arm attributable to entrapment of nerve roots in the intervertebral foramina. The symptoms usually settle with time and treatment is by analgesics in the acute phase. Neck traction is sometimes helpful.
2. *Lumbar spondylosis* (Fig. 118). Degenerative changes in the intervertebral joints of the lumbar spine. Acute exacerbations of pain and stiffness are treated symptomatically.
3. *Spinal stenosis.* Osteophytes on osteoarthritic interfacetal joints may encroach upon the vertebral canal and narrow it. The patient may then develop claudication-like symptoms with a normal peripheral circulation. The diagnosis is confirmed by myelography which shows blockage of the free movement of the radio-opaque medium (Fig. 119). Laminectomy to decompress the vertebral canal may be necessary.
4. *Ankylosing vertebral hyperostosis* (Forestier's disease). Large bony outgrowths arise from the anterior part of the vertebrae at multiple levels (Fig. 120), particularly in the thoracic spine. Stiffness and discomfort are often slight and are treated symptomatically.

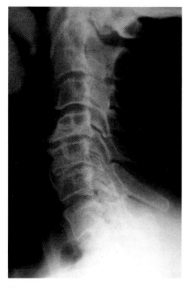

Fig. 117 Cervical spondylosis.

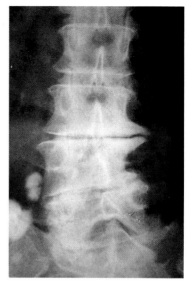

Fig. 118 Lumbar spondylosis.

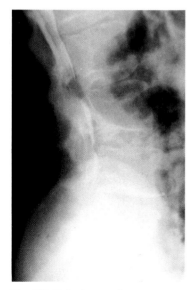

Fig. 119 Spinal stenosis.

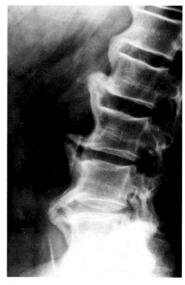

Fig. 120 Ankylosing vertebral hyperostosis.

Congenital high scapula (Sprengel's shoulder)

The scapula develops in the embryo opposite the 4th, 5th and 6th cervical vertebrae and migrates to its usual thoracic position between the 9th and 12th weeks of intrauterine life. Failure of descent causes the deformity in which there is an ugly asymmetry in the line of the shoulders (Fig. 121) and limitation of movements, especially abduction.

The cause is unknown but there is often an abnormal band of fibrous tissue, cartilage or bone connecting the superior angle of the scapula to the cervical spine. Associated congenital anomalies are common.

Treatment

Function of the shoulder is often good, but both appearance and function can be improved by surgical correction.

Frozen shoulder (adhesive capsulitis)

Loss of glenohumeral movement that may be secondary to injury, minor inflammatory conditions, immobilisation of the arm or of idiopathic origin.

Clinical features

Usually unilateral. Middle-aged most often affected. Night pain is a prominent feature. There is loss of both active (Fig. 122) and passive glenohumeral movements.

Treatment

Anti-inflammatory analgesics. Physiotherapy is contraindicated in the early painful phase. The condition is self-limiting but may take up to two years to resolve.

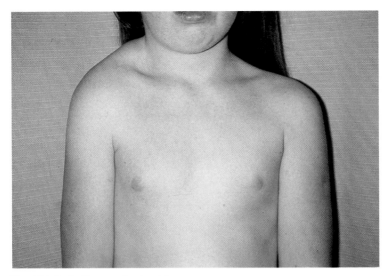

Fig. 121 Right Sprengel's shoulder.

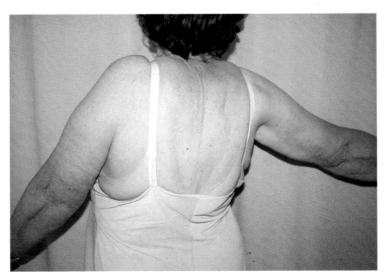

Fig. 122 Frozen left shoulder. Loss of active glenohumeral movement.

Rupture of long head of biceps

Usually a spontaneous rupture without significant stress. Probably caused by degenerative changes in the tendon.

Clinical features

Most common in middle-aged men. Patient may feel that 'something has given way' around the shoulder but pain and functional disability are slight.
The muscle belly displaces distally and looks abnormal when the elbow is flexed against resistance (Fig. 123).

Treatment

Reassurance and normal use.

Acute calcific tendonitis

A not uncommon condition in which periarticular inflammation is associated with the formation of calcium deposits. The shoulder is the joint that is most often involved. Cause unknown.

Clinical features

People in their 30s and 40s are most often affected. The pain is acute in onset and very severe. The joint may be hot and tender. Discomfort settles rapidly over a few days but the condition can recur, or affect the other shoulder. Radiographs will show a typical deposit of calcium (Fig. 124), although this may not be visible early in the attack.

Treatment

Strong analgesics and anti-inflammatory drugs. Aspiration or removal of the calcific deposit may shorten the attack.

Tear of rotator cuff

Acute rupture of the supraspinatus tendon is usually due to age-related degenerative changes in the tendon.

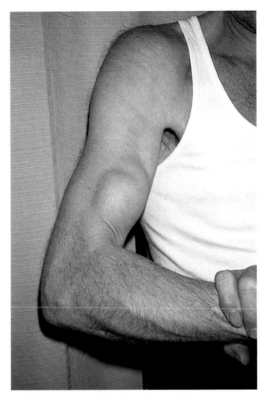

Fig. 123 Rupture of the long head of biceps.

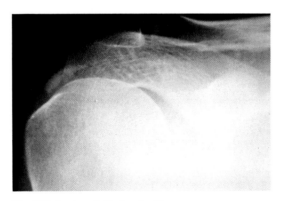

Fig. 124 Acute calcific tendonitis.

Tear of rotator cuff (contd)

Clinical features

Most common in elderly men. After a fall on the shoulder or a sudden strain there is inability to abduct the shoulder actively at the glenohumeral joint. Passive abduction is full (compare with frozen shoulder, p. 81).

X-ray examination is negative, but in long-standing cases the head of the humerus may migrate proximally and impinge on the acromion (Fig. 125).

Treatment

Early surgical repair is indicated in active patients. In the very elderly the tendon is degenerate and difficult to repair; conservative treatment by physiotherapy to keep the shoulder mobile is preferable.

Winging of scapula

The scapula is stabilised on the chest wall by the action of the serratus anterior muscle, innervated by the long thoracic nerve arising from the C5, 6 and 7 roots. Damage to the nerve in its long course may result in paralysis of the serratus anterior muscle and winging of the scapula (Fig. 126). In many cases there is no history of trauma and it is thought that the nerve is affected by a viral mononeuritis.

Clinical features

Paralysis is noted about two weeks after an acute attack of pain in the shoulder. In the similar condition of *neuralgic amyotrophy* there may be more extensive paralysis and wasting of muscles around the shoulder. Young men are most commonly affected, and the right shoulder more than the left.

Treatment

Spontaneous recovery is usual, but may take up to two years.

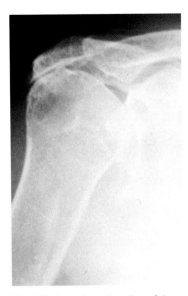

Fig. 125 Superior migration of the head of the humerus after a tear of the rotator cuff.

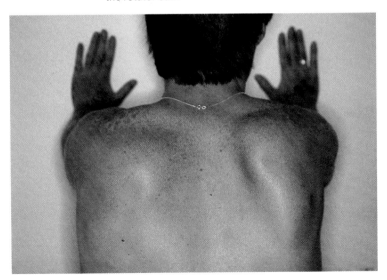

Fig. 126 Winging of the right scapula.

Tennis elbow (epicondylitis)

Discomfort over the lateral epicondyle of the humerus (Fig. 127). Very common.

Cause

The pathology of the lesion is obscure but tearing or degeneration of tendinous tissue has been postulated. Not particularly common in tennis players—more often seen in housewives and repetitive manual work may be a factor.

Clinical features

Apart from tenderness over the lateral epicondyle examination is negative. An 'atypical tennis elbow' with discomfort over the extensor muscle mass may be caused by entrapment of the posterior interosseous nerve in the supinator muscle.

Treatment

Essentially symptomatic by:
1. Local cortisone injection
2. Tennis elbow support—a strap around the forearm just distal to the elbow
3. Surgical release is indicated when there is evidence of posterior interosseous nerve entrapment, not for the typical tennis elbow.

Olecranon bursitis

Inflammatory swelling of the bursa over the olecranon. May be infective or traumatic in origin.

Clinical features

The swelling is obvious (Fig. 128). It is soft and attached to underlying bone.

Treatment

Infected. Antibiotics.   Surgical drainage may be needed.
Traumatic.   Local steroid injection may help the bursitis to resolve.
Excision of the bursa may be followed by slow skin healing.

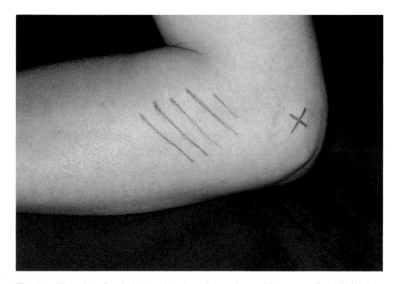

Fig. 127 The site of pain in tennis elbow is marked with a cross. Pain is felt in the hatched area when there is entrapment of the posterior interosseous nerve.

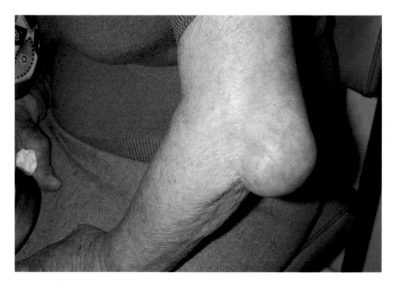

Fig. 128 Olecranon bursitis.

Carpal tunnel syndrome

A common condition in which there is compression of the median nerve beneath the flexor retinaculum at the wrist.

Cause

Usually idiopathic but may be caused by any condition that alters the space in the carpal tunnel, e.g. rheumatoid arthritis (proliferating synovium), pregnancy and hypothyroidism (fluid retention), abnormal muscle bellies and ganglia.

Clinical features

The patient, who is typically a middle-aged woman, is woken during the night with burning or bursting discomfort in the hand. Discomfort is not always confined to the median nerve distribution; often the whole hand and forearm are affected. Relief is obtained by some activity such as shaking the hand, running cold water over it, or getting up and making tea. The hand may feel heavy and numb in the morning. Examination often shows no abnormality. Only in advanced cases is median nerve paresis (p. 103) detectable clinically. Unforced flexion of the wrist for about one minute reproduces the symptoms in about 75% of patients (Phalen's test, Fig. 129).

Treatment

Conservative. Splinting the wrist will often give symptomatic relief.
Diuretics.
Cortisone injection beneath the carpal tunnel.
Surgical. Decompression of the carpal tunnel. A visible constriction in the median nerve (Fig. 130) is not always found.

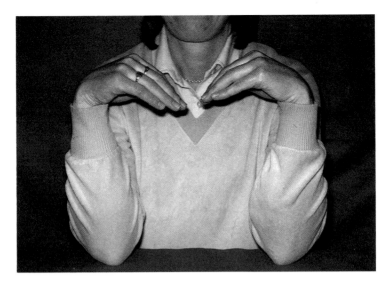

Fig. 129 Phalen's test.

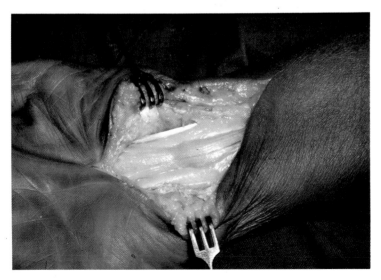

Fig. 130 Decompression of the carpal tunnel. There is a marked constriction in the median nerve.

Kienböck's disease (avascular necrosis of the lunate bone)

Collapse of the bone (Fig. 131) which may be secondary to interference with the blood supply due to trauma.

Clinical features   Affects young adults. Usually there is diffuse wrist pain but the condition may be asymptomatic.

Treatment   *Early stage.*   Rest in plaster.
Late stage.   If secondary symptomatic osteoarthritis occurs the bone can be replaced by a silicone rubber prosthesis. In severe cases arthrodesis of the wrist may be needed.

De Quervain's tenosynovitis

Thickening of the fibrous sheath of the first dorsal compartment of the wrist, which contains the tendons of extensor pollicis brevis and abductor pollicis longus.

Cause   Uncertain, but repetitive movements may aggravate the condition.

Clinical features   Most common in middle-aged women.
There is pain and swelling over the radial styloid process. Discomfort aggravated by ulnar deviation of the wrist, especially when the thumb is gripped (Finkelstein's test, Fig. 132).

Treatment   *Conservative.*   Rest in plaster. Injection of cortisone into sheath.
Surgical.   Release of tendon sheath. All compartments must be released and damage to the terminal branches of the radial nerve avoided, otherwise a troublesome neuroma may form.

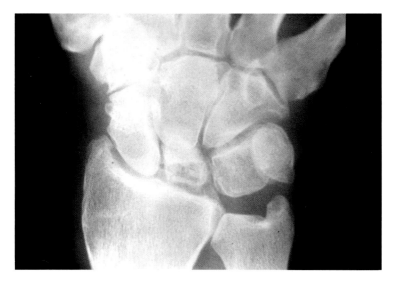

Fig. 131 Avascular necrosis of the lunate bone.

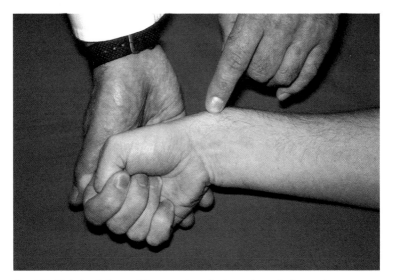

Fig. 132 Finkelstein's test. The examiner deviates the wrist in an ulnar direction.

Congenital anomalies

Classification

1. Failure of formation
2. Failure of separation
3. Duplication
4. Overgrowth
5. Associated with skeletal dysplasias
6. Miscellaneous.

Cause

There may be a clear pattern of inheritance of there may be a non-heritable extrinsic cause (e.g. effect of thalidomide). The hand deformity may be isolated, or associated with other congenital anomalies.

Treatment

May not be necessary. Should be directed to improving function rather than cosmesis. Major reconstructive procedures should be completed before school age if possible. A few representative examples will be illustrated.

Failure of formation
May be transverse or longitudinal.
The commonest level of a transverse defect is the upper third of the forearm (Fig. 133). The deformity is not inherited and treatment is by early fitting of a prosthesis. In longitudinal defects there may be absence or hypoplasia of a digit, for example the thumb (Fig. 134). Distal radial deficiency causes the 'radial club hand' (Fig. 135), which is sporadic in occurrence; it was one of the typical deformities caused by taking thalidomide in early pregnancy.

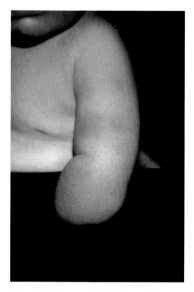

Fig. 133 Congenital defect of the forearm.

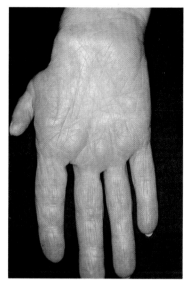

Fig. 134 Hypoplasia of the thumb.

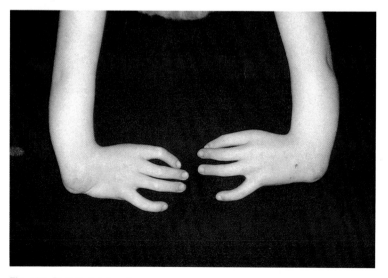

Fig. 135 Radial club hands.

Congenital anomalies (contd)

Failure of separation
One example would be syndactyly (incomplete separation of digits) which may be an isolated abnormality or associated with a generalised disorder.
Inheritance is variable.
In simple syndactyly the fingers are joined by skin alone (Fig. 136); surgical treatment produces a good cosmetic and functional result. In complex syndactyly the fingers are joined by soft tissues and bone; surgical treatment is difficult but worthwhile.

Duplication
The possession of extra digits (polydactyly) is a fairly common example. Inheritance is variable. An obviously abnormal and functionless digit can be removed.

Overgrowth
Isolated gigantism of a digit (macrodactyly) (Fig. 137) may be a feature of neurofibromatosis (p. 43).

Associated with skeletal dysplasias
The hand may be oddly shaped in achondroplasia, the mucopolysaccharidoses (p. 35) and in Marfan's syndrome (p. 45).

Miscellaneous
There are many hand deformities that cannot be classified in the above groups; a typical example is the condition of camptodactyly, a congenital flexion contracture of the proximal interphalangeal joints most often affecting the little fingers (Fig. 138). Usually autosomal dominant inheritance. Function is satisfactory and treatment is rarely needed.

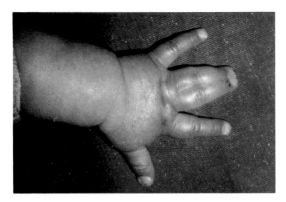

Fig. 136 Syndactyly.

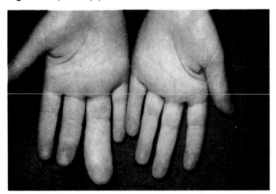

Fig. 137 Macrodactyly.

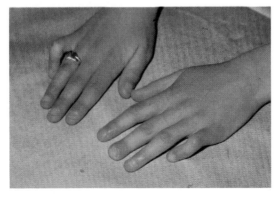

Fig. 138 Camptodactyly.

Ganglion

A cystic swelling associated with joints or synovial tendon sheaths. It consists of a fibrous capsule containing viscous fluid and may be caused by a herniation of synovial tissues.

Clinical features

Most commonly found on the dorsoradial aspect of the wrist in young adults (Fig. 139). Sometimes associated with discomfort, but often symptomless.

Treatment

About 50% disappear spontaneously. Excision is only indicated if the ganglion is large or causing significant symptoms, e.g. by pressing on a nerve.

Pigmented villonodular synovitis (giant cell tumour of tendon sheath; benign synovioma)

A lobular tumour, probably of synovial origin, arising from joints and tendon sheaths. Often has yellowish appearance on section, because it contains lipid and haemosiderin; giant cells are not always present.

Clinical features

Most common in middle age. Presents as a painless firm swelling on the flexor aspect of a finger or arising from the distal joint (Fig. 140). Sometimes larger joints such as the knee are affected.

Treatment

Excision. May recur if excision is incomplete.

Implantation dermoid

A subcutaneous nodule due to implantation of skin cells by a penetrating injury. Almost invariably found on the flexor aspect of the hand (Fig. 141).

Treatment

Excision.

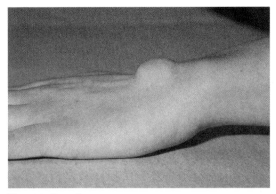

Fig. 139 Ganglion.

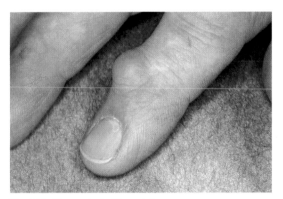

Fig. 140 Pigmented villonodular synovitis.

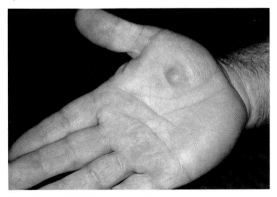

Fig. 141 Implantation dermoid.

Trigger finger (stenosing tenosynovitis; locking finger)

A common condition in which the finger or thumb cannot be actively straightened from the flexed position.

Cause

There is a disparity in size between the flexor tendons and the mouth of the fibrous flexor sheath. Sometimes a nodule forms on the tendon, which can be withdrawn from the tendon sheath by the action of the powerful flexor muscles but tends to stick in the mouth of the sheath when the hand relaxes, thus preventing full extension of the digit. Usually spontaneous in onset, but may be aggravated by repetitive movements. Common in diabetics and patients with rheumatoid arthritis who may have flexor tendon synovitis (p. 11).

Clinical features

Most common in the middle-aged, although congenital flexion deformity of the thumb due to the same mechanism is sometimes seen in infants and young children (Fig. 142). Adult patients complain of 'sticking' or 'locking' of a finger or thumb, and have to straighten the digit passively (Fig. 143). Pain on straightening the digit may be referred to the proximal interphalangeal joint.

Treatment

Injection of hydrocortisone around the tendon at the mouth of the fibrous flexor sheath.
Surgical release of the mouth of the sheath if injection fails.

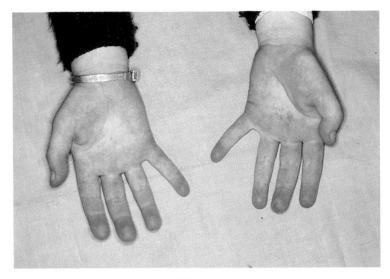

Fig. 142 Left trigger thumb in a child.

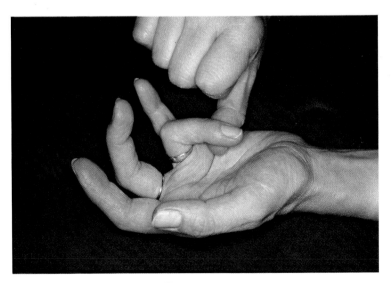

Fig. 143 Straightening a trigger finger.

Dupuytren's disease

A common condition in which the palmar and digital fascia become thickened and sometimes contracted.

Cause

Unknown. Common in people of European descent but very rare in other races. There is a strong hereditary element; the condition appears to be transmitted as an autosomal dominant with variable penetrance.

Often attributed to previous injury or heavy manual work, but just as common in people with sedentary jobs.

Pathology

Aggregates of contractile fibroblasts form within the fibrous palmar and digital fascia.

Clinical features

Usually occurs in middle and old age. The earliest stage is thickening and nodularity of the palmar fascia without contracture (Fig. 144). Knuckle pads (Garrod's pads, Fig. 145) sometimes form on the dorsum of the proximal interphalangeal joints, although they also occur without other features of Dupuytren's disease being present. In some patients the nodularity progresses to form contracted cords passing into the fingers; the ulnar side of the hand is most often involved (Fig. 146). Secondary contractures of the capsule of the proximal interphalangeal joints may occur.

Treatment

Depends on severity and extent of the disease. Surgery is indicated for early progressive contractures and established deformity. The operation of choice is removal of the abnormal fascia (local fasciectomy); it should be done before secondary capsular contractures have become established.

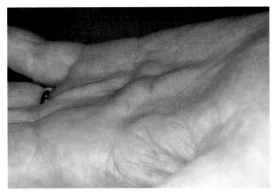

Fig. 144 Dupuytren's tissue in the palm of the hand.

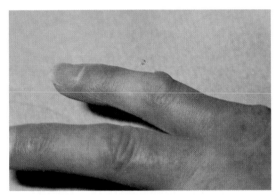

Fig. 145 Knuckle pad on little finger.

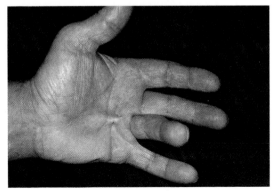

Fig. 146 Typical contracture affecting the ring finger.

Nerve lesions

The hand is supplied by the median, ulnar and radial nerves. The radial nerve supplies sensation to the dorsoradial surface of the hand and loss of radial nerve sensation is not disabling in the hand.

Nerves may be divided in any open injury of the hand or forearm. Surgical repair should be performed by an expert. Full recovery is not always achieved in mixed motor and sensory nerves in adults, but useful functional recovery is gained in many cases.

Median nerve
Motor   to abductor pollicis brevis, opponens pollicis, part or all of flexor pollicis brevis and the radial two lumbricals in the hand. In the forearm it supplies all the flexor muscles with the exception of flexor carpi ulnaris and the ulnar half of flexor digitorum profundus.

Sensory   to skin over the thenar eminence and palmar surface of the thumb and the radial two and one half fingers.

(Variations in the motor and sensory distributions are not uncommon.)

Loss of function in the median nerve results in inability to abduct the thumb (Fig. 147). Wasting of the thenar muscles will follow (Fig. 148). When the median nerve is damaged proximally in the arm there is loss of active flexion of the index finger; the other fingers can be flexed by the action of the ulnar innervated portion of flexor digitorum profundus (Fig. 149).

See also carpal tunnel syndrome, p. 89.

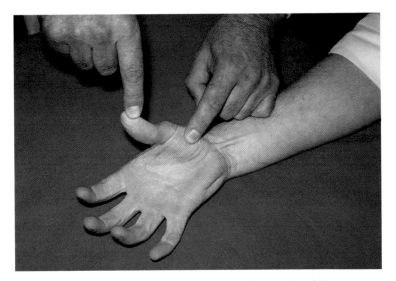

Fig. 147 Testing normal abduction of the thumb. Contraction of the muscle is visible and palpable.

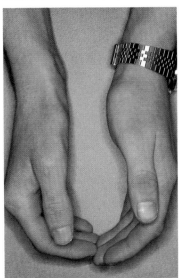

Fig. 148 Wasting of the thenar muscles in the right hand.

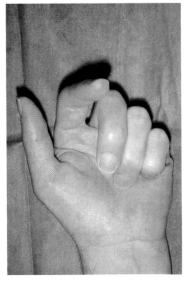

Fig. 149 Attempted flexion of the fingers produces the 'sign of benediction' when there is a proximal lesion of the median nerve.

Nerve lesions (contd)

Ulnar nerve
Motor to the intrinsic muscles of the hand that are not supplied by the median nerve.
Sensory to the palmar aspect of the ulnar one and a half fingers and the whole of the back of the hand except for the area supplied by the radial nerve.

Damage to the ulnar nerve leads to wasting of the intrinsic muscles, most obviously the first dorsal interosseous, and the little and ring fingers adopt a position of slight flextion—the 'ulnar claw hand' (Fig. 150). Clawing is more marked when the ulnar nerve is damaged at the wrist.

Froment's sign. When the patient attempts to grip a flat object between the thumb and the hand the flexor pollicis longus muscle (innervated by the median nerve) comes into play because the adductor pollicis muscle is paralysed; hence the thumb on the affected side flexes at the interphalangeal joint (Fig. 151).

Loss of function in the ulnar nerve is not as disabling as loss of the median nerve. There is some loss of dexterity and weakness of grip but function is often surprisingly good.

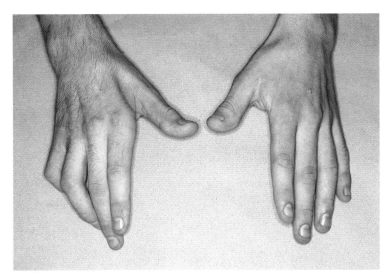

Fig. 150 Ulnar paralysis. Note wasting of the first dorsal interosseous muscle.

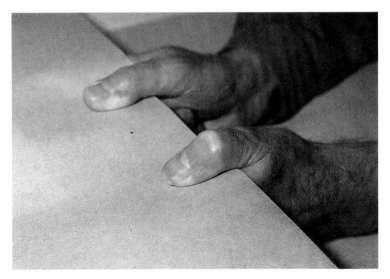

Fig. 151 Positive Froment's sign in the left hand.

Osteoarthritis

For a general description of OA, see p. 7. Although OA typically affects major weight bearing joints such as the hip and knee, it is not uncommon in the hand.

Clinical features

The characteristic feature of OA in the hands is involvement of the distal interphalangeal joints, producing Heberden's notes which are due to osteophytes around the joint (Fig. 152). Sometimes a cystic lesion which is similar in nature to a ganglion (p. 97) may arise from the distal interphalangeal joint; this so-called 'mucous cyst' (Fig. 152) can cause grooving of the nail. The carpometacarpal joint of the thumb is often affected by OA (Fig. 153). The patient has pain on gripping, or wringing out clothes. An adduction contracture of thumb may occur (Fig. 154).

Treatment

Involvement of the distal interphalangeal joints seldom requires surgical treatment, although removal of unsightly mucous cysts is sometimes requested. Recurrence of mucous cyst is common unless care is taken to obtain good skin cover of the joint after excision.

Carpometacarpal OA affecting the thumb is ofter disabling; if it does not respond to conservative treatment by rest and anti-inflammatory analgesic drugs, surgical treatment by arthrodesis or arthroplasty of the joint may be necessary.

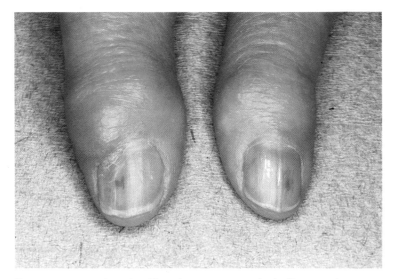

Fig. 152 Heberden's nodes. There is a mucous cyst in the finger on the left.

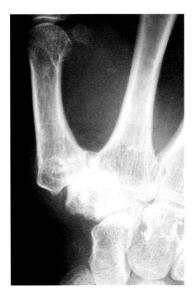

Fig. 153 Osteoarthritis of the carpometacarpal joint of the thumb.

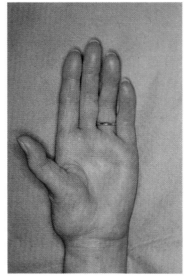

Fig. 154 Typical thumb deformity in carpometacarpal OA.

Congenital dislocation of the hip (CDH)

Occurs in about 3 – 5/1000 new-born children in Britain, but varies considerably between countries and races (e.g. almost unknown in Bantu).

Cause

Unknown. Commoner in females, first born and after breech delivery. May be a family history.

Clinical features

Early. All new-born children should be screened for CDH. The flexed hips are abducted; if a hip is dislocated it will usually slip back into the acetabulum with a palpable 'clunk' during this manoeuvre (Ortolani's test, Fig. 155). The test should be done when the child is relaxed after a feed. Radiographs are difficult to interpret because the hip is largely cartilaginous.
Late. Unless detected in the neonatal period the diagnosis is seldom made before the child begins to walk, when a limp and leg length discrepancy may be apparent. Radiographs confirm the diagnosis (Fig. 156).

Treatment

Early. The hips should be splinted in flexion and abduction until they are stable; treatment should begin in the neonatal period for best results.
Late. Treatment becomes considerably more difficult as the child gets older. Open reduction and surgical reorientation of the acetabulum and femoral head are usually necessary. Early degenerative arthritis is liable to occur unless the hip is completely congruent.

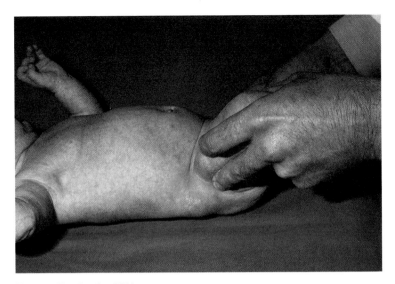

Fig. 155 Testing for CDH.

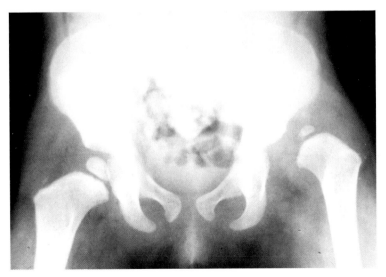

Fig. 156 Untreated CDH in a child.

Femoral anteversion

The angle of anterversion lies between the axis of the head and neck of the femur and the plane of the front of the femoral condyles. If this angle is large the range of internal rotation at the hips will be greater than normal (Fig. 157) and the range of external rotation correspondingly diminished.

Clinical features

Children with marked femoral anteversion often walk with their feet and patellae turned inward (Fig. 158); this 'hen-toed' gait is a cause of parental concern. When sitting the child favours the 'W' position (Fig. 159); this is probably a result rather than a cause of the anterversion.

Treatment

Spontaneous improvement almost always occurs without specific treatment by the age of 10. There is seldom any disability in children in whom full correction does not occur. The condition should be regarded as a variation of normal development, rather than a pathological disorder, and the parents reassured.

Intoeing gait due to femoral anteversion should be distinguished from intoeing due to metatarsus adductus (p. 135). Intoeing may also be caused by mild genu valgum ('knock knees') since the feet are turned inwards to provide a stable base for walking.

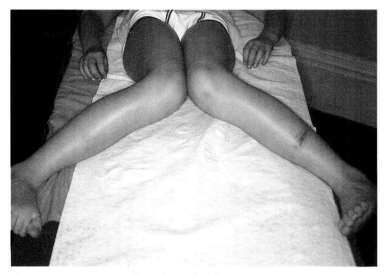

Fig. 157 Increased internal rotation at the hips.

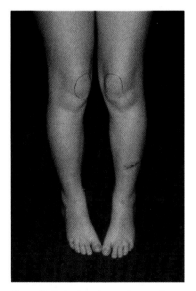

Fig. 158 Intoeing due to femoral anteversion.

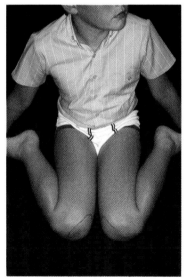

Fig. 159 The 'W' position.

Perthes' disease (coxa plana)

Collapse and later regeneration of the ossific centre of the head of the femur.

Cause

Unknown, but thought to be due to a disturbance in blood supply to the head of the femur.

Clinical features

Affects children aged 4–10. The child may be noticed to limp or complain of pain in the groin or the inner aspect of the knee. On examination in the acute phase there is usually limitation of movements of the hip and visible muscle spasm on passive rotation of the extended hip (Fig. 160).

Investigations

Radiographs show collapse and fragmentation of the ossific centre (Fig. 161).

Progress

Recovery takes about two years and the extent of recovery is very variable. Some children show full recovery without treatment, others develop progressive deformity of the femoral head and osteoarthritis of the hip in early adult life. Some idea of the prognosis can be gained from the extent of changes in the head of the femur on initial radiographs.

Treatment

Traction while there is muscle spasm. Weight bearing should be avoided until hip movements are full.
Femoral or pelvic osteotomy may be indicated in some children to prevent progressive deformity of the femoral head, but results are unpredictable.

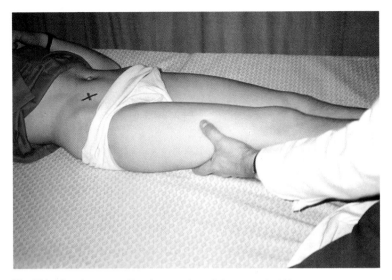

Fig. 160 Muscle spasm. Passive rotation of the extended hip causes involuntary contraction of the abdominal muscles.

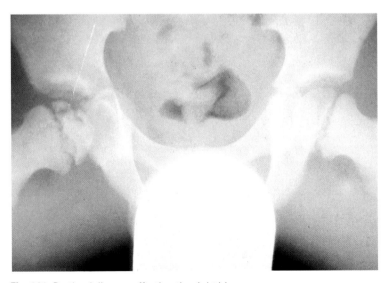

Fig. 161 Perthes' disease affecting the right hip.

Hip (4)

Slipped upper femoral epiphysis (adolescent coxa vara)

A posteroinferior displacement of the proximal femoral epiphysis, occurring in the absence of major injury. Cause unknown, but 50% of children affected have an abnormality of body build, either obesity or extreme slenderness, and a hormonal effect on the growth plate may be involved.

Clinical features

Occurs in 10 – 18 age group. There is gradual onset of a limp and pain in the hip or knee. The displacement happens gradually but may be accelerated by falls at sports or games. On examination there is limitation of abduction and medial rotation of the hip and the leg lies in external rotation if the slip is severe. An early slip is easily missed on AP films of the hip (Fig. 162) but is much more clearly seen on lateral films taken with the hips in the 'frog' position, and these should always be done (Fig. 163). A complete slip is unmistakable (Fig. 164). Both hips are affected in 25%.

Treatment

Early slip. The epiphysis should be stabilised with fine pins passed up the neck of the femur as a matter of urgency.
Severe slip. Manipulative reduction is avoided because of the risk of causing avascular necrosis of the head of the femur. The deformity is corrected by open reduction or upper femoral osteotomy.

Complications

Deformity, avascular necrosis, loss of articular cartilage (chondrolysis), secondary arthritis.

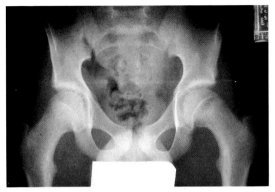

Fig. 162 Early slip of left femoral epiphysis. Anteroposterior view.

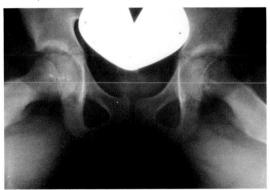

Fig. 163 Early slip of left femoral epiphysis. 'Frog lateral' view with hips flexed and abducted.

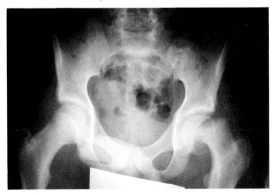

Fig. 164 Severe slip of left femoral epiphysis.

Osteoarthritis

For a general description of OA, p. 7. OA of the hip is a common and disabling condition of middle aged and elderly people.
It may be primary (idiopathic) or secondary to previous injury, Perthes' disease (p. 113), slipped upper femoral epiphysis (p. 115), avascular necrosis (p. 47) and congenital subluxation (partial dislocation) of the hip (p. 109).

Clinical features

Pain, stiffness, loss of movement, deformity and a limp. The commonest deformity is a combined adduction, flexion and external rotation contracture of the hip, often causing an apparent leg length discrepancy. A flexion deformity can be demonstrated by flexing the good hip until the normal lumbar lordosis is obliterated (Thomas' test, Fig. 165). Radiographs show loss of joint space, sclerosis of periarticular bone, osteophytes and cysts (Fig. 166).

Treatment

Mild disability. Analgesics, physiotherapy, use of a stick (in hand opposite affected hip) and weight loss if appropriate.
Severe disability. In young people arthrodesis is the most suitable operation, although it is rarely necessary. Upper femoral osteotomy can be performed at any age if the range of hip movement is good, but the most common procedure in the older patient is total hip replacement (p. 9).

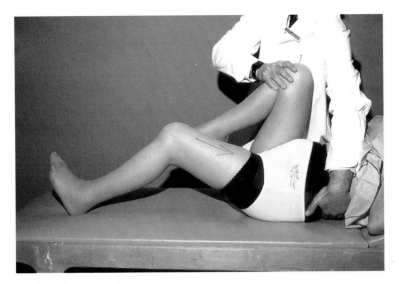

Fig. 165 Thomas' test.

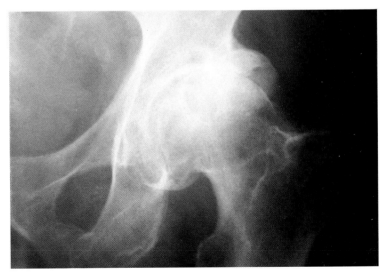

Fig. 166 Osteoarthritis of the hip.

Bursitis

Enlargement of bursae around the knee is a common complaint. Bursitis is usually secondary to chronic irritation (e.g. kneeling) but it may occasionally be infective.

Examples of bursae that are commonly enlarged are the semimembranosus bursa in childhood (Fig. 167) and the prepatellar and infrapatellar bursae (Fig. 168) in adults.

Treatment Irritative bursitis usually settles without treatment if the cause is avoided; infected bursae may need drainage and antibiotic treatment.

Baker's cyst

A synovial herniation into the popliteal fossa (Fig. 169).

Usually secondary to some intra-articular problem such as osteoarthritis (p. 129) or a degenerate meniscus, particularly if the underlying condition is associated with a chronic synovial effusion.

Occasionally the cyst ruptures and synovial fluid tracks into the calf muscles, mimicking a deep venous thrombosis.

Treatment Excision of the cyst is seldom indicated unless the underlying condition can be treated, as otherwise recurrence is almost the rule.

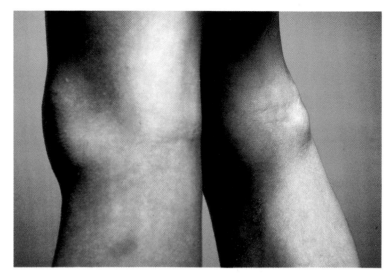

Fig. 167 An enlarged semimembranosus bursa in the right knee.

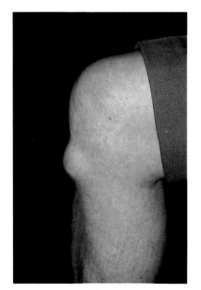

Fig. 168 Infrapatellar bursitis.

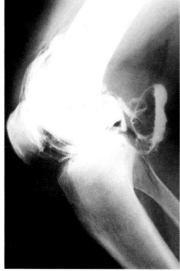

Fig. 169 Arthrogram showing a Baker's cyst.

Disorders of the menisci

Acute tears. Commonly caused by twisting injuries. Medial meniscus is damaged more often than the lateral; it may tear to form a tag (Fig. 170) or a longitudinal split (a 'bucket handle'). The torn part of the meniscus can displace between the femoral and tibial condyles, causing sudden inability to extend the knee ('locking'). Recurrent effusions are common.

When the history is doubtful, inspection of the interior of the knee through an arthroscope (Fig. 171) can be helpful. The menisci can also be delineated by arthrography.

Treatment is by partial or complete removal of the affected meniscus.

Degenerative tears. Common in the middle-aged and elderly. May cause aching discomfort and sometimes an effusion. Locking is not a symptom as the tear lies horizontally within the meniscus and displacement does not occur. Symptoms often settle spontaneously and meniscectomy should be avoided if possible as it may accelerate degenerative changes in articular cartilage.

Meniscal cysts. May be associated with degenerative changes within a meniscus, usually the lateral meniscus. There is a tense swelling on the joint line (Fig. 172) and aching discomfort. Treatment is by excision of the cyst plus meniscectomy if the meniscus is clearly abnormal.

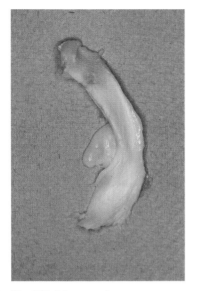

Fig. 170 A torn meniscus.

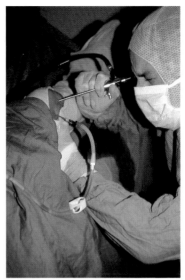

Fig. 171 Arthroscopy.

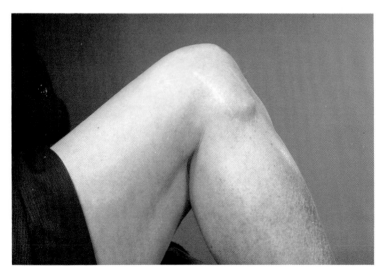

Fig. 172 A cyst of the lateral meniscus.

Tibial apophysitis (Osgood–Schlatter's disease)

Enlargement and fragmentation of the tibial tuberosity.

Clinical features

Common in boys around 12 – 14 years. The complaint is of pain over the tibial tuberosity which is visibly and palpably enlarged (Fig. 173). Discomfort is often aggravated by activity. Radiographs show some fragmentation of the apophysis (Fig. 174).

Treatment

Most do not need treatment but if the knee is painful on strenuous exercise it is sensible to restrict athletic pursuits. The condition is self-limiting and the long-term function of the knee is normal. Very occasionally a small separate ossicle may remain after the apophysis has fused, and may warrant excision.

Calcification in the medial collateral ligament (Pellegrini–Stieda's disease)

This condition can occur after a partial tear of the proximal part of the medial collateral ligament.

Clinical features

Local swelling and discomfort. Radiographs (Fig. 175) confirm the diagnosis.

Treatment

Local anaesthetic and corticosteroid injection.

A similar picture is seen in acute calcific tendonitis (p. 83) around the knee, but the onset is usually more acute and there is no history of injury. The treatment is the same.

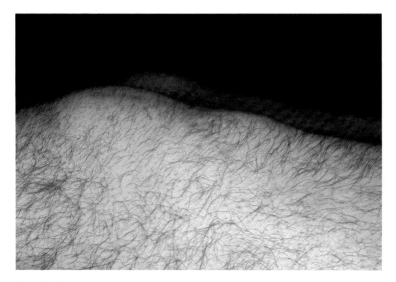

Fig. 173 Tibial apophysitis.

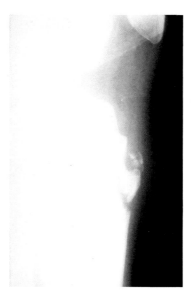

Fig. 174 Tibial apophysitis.

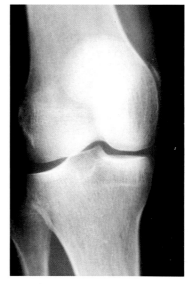

Fig. 175 Calcification in the medial collateral ligament.

Chondromalacia patellae

Retropatellar knee pain is extremely common in teenaged girls and is occasionally attributable to changes in the articular cartilage of the patellae (Fig. 176), although often no cause is found.

Clinical features

Discomfort, often worse on stairs. Clinical examination often negative although there may be joint laxity and moderate genu valgum. Radiographs are normal. Arthroscopy will reveal changes in the cartilage, if present.

Treatment

Analgesics: soluble aspirin seems to be most effective.
Restriction of activities may be necessary. Various operations have been described for this condition but the results are unpredictable and frequently disappointing.

Recurrent subluxation of the patella

Clinical features

Most common in teenaged girls and young women. Subluxation occurs in a lateral direction and the knee suddenly gives way, causing the patient to fall to the ground.
On examination there may be mild joint laxity, genu valgum and often a small, high patella. The patient is apprehensive when the patella is pushed laterally.
Tangential radiographs usually show hypoplasia of the lateral femoral condyle and incongruity of the patellofemoral articulation (Fig. 177).

Treatment

Physiotherapy to develop the quadriceps muscle. Surgical repositioning of the patella if symptoms persist.

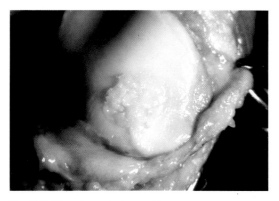

Fig. 176 Chondromalacia patellae.

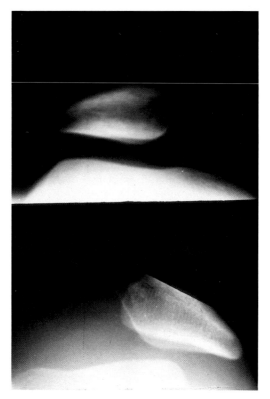

Fig. 177 Subluxation of the patella. The other
knee is shown above for comparison.

Osteochondritis dissecans

Separation of an avascular fragment of bone and cartilage from the surface of a joint. Medial femoral condyle is most often affected (Fig. 178). Cause unknown, but may have a traumatic basis.

Clinical features

Usually affects boys aged 10–18. The initial complaint is local discomfort, but if the fragment separates it may become trapped between the joint surfaces, causing sudden locking (Fig. 179). Secondary osteoarthritis can affect the joint in early adult life.

Treatment

Before separation. The fragment may heal back into place with rest. Drilling the bone may encourage revascularisation.
After separation. It may be possible to pin the fragment back into place but if not it should be removed.

Blount's disease (tibia vara)

An uncommon condition in which there is abnormal growth of the medial part of the proximal tibial epiphysis. Cause unknown; similar deformities can occur after injury or infection.

Clinical features

West Indian children are most often affected.
Infantile type. Accentuation of the normal bow-legged appearance of the toddler, progressing to a severe deformity in later childhood. The varus deformity is associated with an internal rotational deformity of the tibia.
Adolescent type. Unilateral, onset age 8–15 (Fig. 180). Final deformity not as severe as infantile type.

Treatment

Correction by osteotomy.

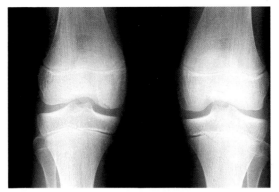

Fig. 178 Early osteochondritis dissecans, right medial femoral condyle.

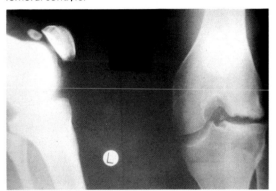

Fig. 179 Irregularity of joint surface and a loose body.

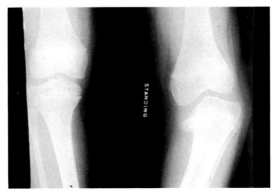

Fig. 180 Blount's disease.

Osteoarthritis

For a general description of osteoarthritis, see p. 7. OA affecting the knee is a very common condition and is usually secondary to some recognisable cause such as obesity, previous injury or previous meniscectomy (Fig. 181).

Clinical features

Often bilateral. The major complaints are of pain and stiffness.

On examination there is often a knee flexion deformity, or genu varum if only the medial compartment of the knee is affected (Fig. 182). Radiographs show the usual features of OA, affecting one or more of the articular areas of the knee.

Treatment

Analgesics, weight loss when appropriate. Surgical treatment may be indicated if the symptoms are not controlled by such measures. Realignment of the tibia by upper tibial osteotomy is often helpful if OA is confined to the medial compartment and there is a varus deformity (Figs. 183, 184). Arthrodesis of the knee is seldom indicated; although it is successful in relieving pain the inability to bend the knee is a serious inconvenience. Total knee replacement is not as successful in patients with OA as it is in patients with knees affected by rheumatoid arthritis; patients with OA are often overweight and quite active, and early loosening of the prosthetic joint can be a serious problem.

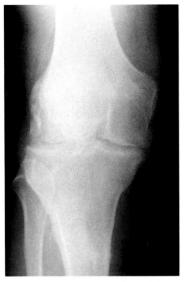

Fig. 181 Osteoarthritis of the right knee, twenty years after medial and lateral meniscectomies.

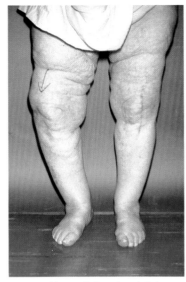

Fig. 182 Varus deformity of right knee.

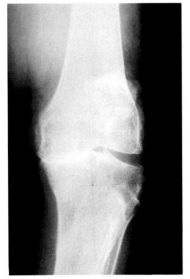

Fig. 183 OA of the medical compartment causing a varus deformity.

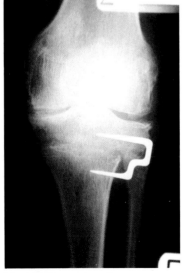

Fig. 184 Correction of varus deformity by upper tibial osteotomy.

Heel bump (winter heel; pump bump)

Prominent thickening over the superolateral border of the calcaneum (Fig. 185). Usually seen in teenaged girls; often bilateral.

Treatment

Pad beneath heel to minimise pressure from back of shoe.
Spontaneous improvement is common and surgical treatment by calcaneal trimming or osteotomy is rarely necessary.

Rupture of calcaneal tendon

May affect athletes or, more commonly, middle-aged people during activities such as dancing. There may be a palpable gap in the tendon. When the calf on the affected side is squeezed the foot fails to plantar flex (Fig. 186).

Treatment

Surgical repair or rest in plaster with the foot in a plantar-flexed position.

Plantar fasciitis

Discomfort beneath the calcaneum at the attachment of the plantar fascia. Sometimes occurs in inflammatory arthropathies, but often no cause is found.
The pain is aggravated by weight bearing. Clinical examination is negative apart from local tenderness. A heel spur (Fig. 187) is often seen on radiographs but is a common normal finding and is of no significance.

Treatment

Doughnut heel pad. Local anaesthetic and steroid injection. Local ultrasound treatment. Condition settles spontaneously, but may take some months to do so.

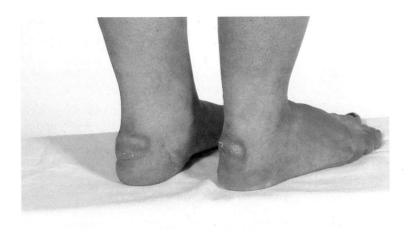

Fig. 185 Heel bumps.

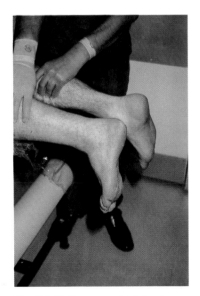

Fig. 186 Calf squeeze test. Rupture of left calcaneal tendon.

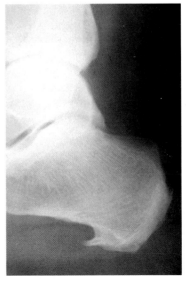

Fig. 187 Heel spur. An incidental finding in plantar fasciitis.

Talipes equinovarus (club foot)

A congenital deformity in which the foot points downwards and is twisted inwards. The cause is unknown, although there may be a family history. A similar deformity can occur in spina bifida and arthrogryphosis (p. 29).

Clinical features

The deformity, which is obvious at birth, may be unilateral or bilateral (Fig. 188). The foot cannot be dorsiflexed to touch the front of the shin and there is often a deep skin crease on the medial border of the sole. (Fig. 189).

Treatment

Neonatal. Treatment should start as soon as possible, because the foot will rapidly stiffen in the position of deformity. The foot is strapped in the corrected position; plaster may be used as the child grows.
Later. If full correction cannot be achieved by strapping, or if there has been no early treatment, surgical release of tight soft tissues will be needed.

Talipes calcaneovalgus

A congenital deformity in which the foot points upwards and is twisted outwards (Fig. 190). Usually attributable to positioning *in utero* but may be caused by neurological disorders such as spina bifida.

Treatment

Unlike talipes equinovarus the deformity improves spontaneously as the child begins to move the legs freely, provided there is no underlying neurological abnormality. Treatment by splintage is seldom needed.

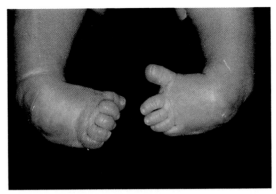

Fig. 188 Talipes equinovarus.

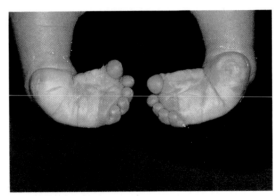

Fig. 189 Talipes equinovarus.

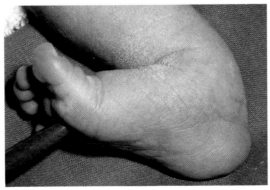

Fig. 190 Talipes calcaneovalgus.

Metatarsus adductus

A common condition in which the anterior part of the foot is deviated medially (Fig. 191) causing the child to walk with an intoeing gait.

Clinical features

Affects children aged 2 – 8. The foot can be passively corrected into the normal position. Physical examination will distinguish between metatarsus adductus and femoral anteversion (p. 111) which also causes an intoeing gait.

Treatment

In the majority of children the appearance improves without active treatment, although it may take some years.

Pes cavus

Accentuation of the longitudinal arch of the foot.

Causes

Idiopathic, familial, or associated with neurological disorders such as poliomyelitis (p. 25), spina bifida (p. 29) and peroneal muscle atrophy (p. 31).

Clinical features

May be unilateral or bilateral, depending on cause. Pes cavus is usually apparent in childhood and is obvious on examination (Fig. 192) Clawing of the toes (p. 143) is almost always present. In older children and adults there may be pain associated with callosities on the toes and under the metatarsal heads.

Treatment

Appropriate footwear.
The foot may be corrected by release of soft tissues in childhood, if the deformity warrants it. In adults it may be necessary to remove a wedge of bone to gain correction. Claw toes can be straightened at the same time.

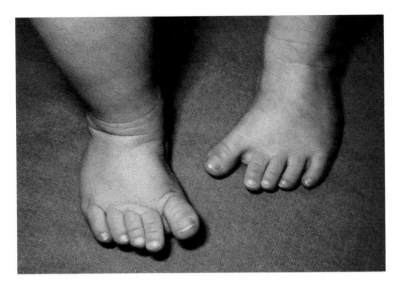

Fig. 191 Metatarsus adductus.

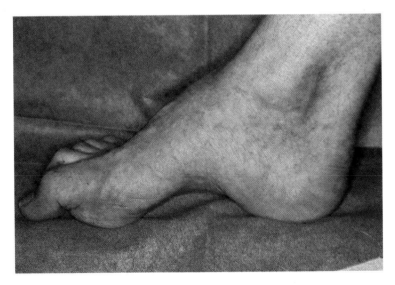

Fig. 192 Pes cavus.

Pes planus (flat foot)

In this common condition the medial border of the foot is in contact with the ground when standing (Fig. 193). Often the whole foot appears to have rotated into eversion around its longitudinal axis. Two main types of flat foot are recognised, as follows.

Mobile flat foot
The longitudinal arch is fully restored when standing on tip-toe. Symptoms are usually absent or mild. There may be some aching discomfort in the foot, and the shoes may wear rapidly on the inner border.

Treatment

An inner arch raise may be helpful symptomatically, but the appearance is usually permanent. Surgical treatment is rarely needed.

Rigid flat foot
The longitudinal arch is not restored when standing on tip-toe. Often caused by a bony bridge (synostosis or bar) between two of the tarsal bones. Talocalcaneal and calcaneonavicular bars (Fig. 194) are most common.
Typically, a youngster around the age of 12 complains of pain in the foot and may be noted to have protective spasm of the peroneal muscles, hence the term 'peroneal spastic flat foot' (Fig. 195).
Radiographs show the bar, but special views may be needed.

Treatment

Resection of the bar if this is feasible. Arthrodesis of the subtalar and midtarsal joints (triple arthrodesis) may be necessary.

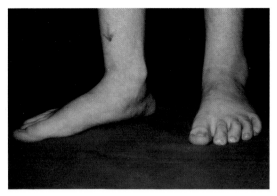

Fig. 193 Flat feet.

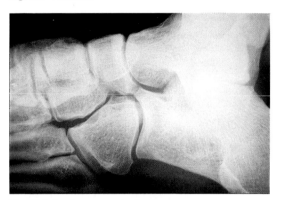

Fig. 194 A calcaneonavicular bar.

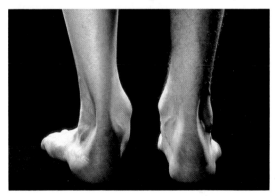

Fig. 195 Peroneal spasm affecting the left foot.

Osteochondritis of the navicular bone (Köhler's disease)

Collapse of the ossific centre of the bone. Like osteochondritis affecting other bones it is thought to be caused by a disturbance in the blood supply.

Clinical features

Affects children aged 3–5. The child may complain of pain and be noticed to limp when walking.
Radiographs show compression and sometimes fragmentation of the ossification centre in the bone (Fig. 196).

Treatment

Resolves spontaneously in a year or two. Rest in a plaster for a few weeks may be necessary if discomfort is severe.

Osteochondritis of a metatarsal bone (Freiberg's infraction)

Deformity of the second (occasionally third) metatarsal head. May be caused by an interruption in the blood supply due to injury.

Clinical features

Affects teenagers. Complaint is of pain on walking. On examination there may be soft tissue thickening around the affected joint. Radiographs confirm the diagnosis (Fig. 197).

Treatment

Indicated only if pain is severe.
Early stages. Rest in plaster.
Late cases. Excision arthroplasty is occasionally indicated for pain due to osteoarthritis.

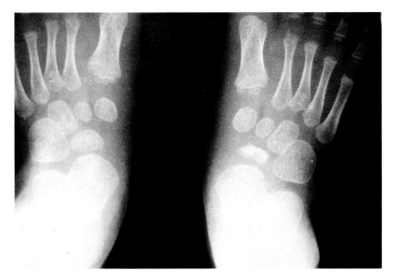

Fig. 196 Osteochondritis of the navicular bone in the right foot.

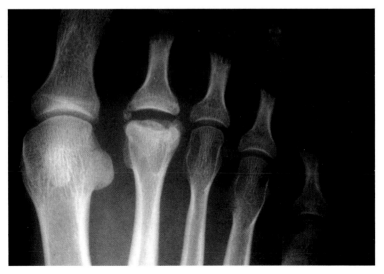

Fig. 197 Osteochondritis of the second metatarsal bone.

17 | Foot (5)

Syndactyly

Like syndactyly in the hand (p. 95), syndactyly in the foot may involve skin alone (Fig. 198) or be complex and associated with multiple digital anomalies.

Treatment

Unlike the hand, the function of the foot is not affected by syndactyly and surgical correction is unlikely to improve the appearance of the foot.

Over-riding of the little toe (digitus quintus varus)

A fairly common congenital anomaly (Fig. 199). The deformity can initially be passively corrected but does not improve spontaneously and may become fixed and subject to pressure from shoes.

Treatment

Surgical correction is usually necessary.

Under-riding toes (curly toes; varus toes)

A varus curvature of the lesser toes, usually most marked in the third and fourth toes (Fig. 200). There is often a family history.
The toes function normally and some spontaneous improvement in the appearance is common.

Treatment

Seldom needed. In severe cases the alignment of the toes can be improved by transferring the flexor tendon into the extensor tendon around the lateral border of the toe.

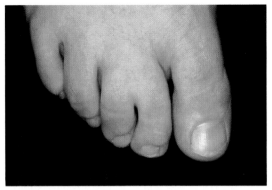

Fig. 198 Syndactyly between second and third toes.

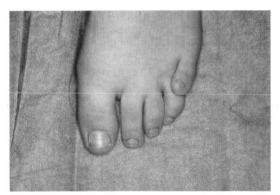

Fig. 199 Over-riding fifth toe.

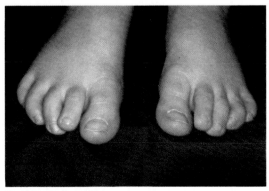

Fig. 200 Under-riding toes.

Hammer toe

Fixed flexion of the proximal interphalangeal joint of one of the lesser toes (Fig. 201). May occur as an isolated deformity, or be associated with hallux valgus (p. 145). A painful callosity often forms on the dorsum of the affected joint.

Treatment

Local pads to relieve pressure or arthrodesis of the affected joint in a straight position.

Mallet toe

Fixed flexion of the terminal interphalangeal joint of one of the lesser toes (Fig. 202). A painful callosity often forms on the pulp of the affected toe.

Treatment

As for hammer toe (see above).

Claw toes

Flexion of the interphalangeal joints and extension of the metatarsophalangeal joints of one or, more commonly, several of the lesser toes (Fig. 203). Caused by an imbalance of the intrinsic and extrinsic muscles acting on the toes. Often found in association with pes cavus (p. 135). May be idiopathic or caused by any condition interfering with muscle function in the foot, e.g. spina bifida (p. 29), poliomyelitis (p. 25), peroneal muscle atrophy (p. 31) and ischaemia.

Treatment

Shoes should have plenty of room for the toes. Surgical correction is by tendon transfers if the deformity is mobile, or arthrodesis if it is fixed.

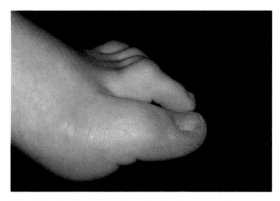

Fig. 201 Hammer toe deformity in the second toe.

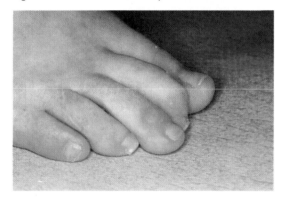

Fig. 202 Mallet toe deformity in the second toe.

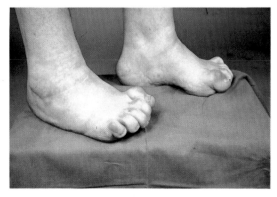

Fig. 203 Clawing of toes.

Hallux valgus

The great toe is excessively deviated towards the second toe and indeed may come to lie over or under it.

Cause

Unknown. Often a strong family history. Wearing tight pointed shoes may aggravate the deformity but probably does not cause it.

Clinical features

A common condition in middle-aged and elderly women. The patient complains of pressure over the head of the first metatarsal bone or over the second toe (Fig. 204). An inflamed bursa may form over the first metatarsal head. Shoe fitting is a problem. There may be spreading of the metatarsal heads, causing widening of the foot and often a painful callosity forms under the second metatarsal head (Fig. 206). Radiographs confirm the deformity (Fig. 205). Sometimes the second toe is dislocated at the metatarsophalangeal joint.

Treatment

Conservative. Comfortable shoes. Protection of pressure areas.
Surgical. Many operations have been described. In young people the great toe can be realigned by osteotomy of the first metatarsal. In older patients arthrodesis or excisional arthroplasty (Keller's arthroplasty) of the first metatarsophalangeal joint are preferred. The results of operation for this condition are often disappointing in the long-term. Realigning the big toe will not relieve pain from plantar callosities, which is often the major complaint.

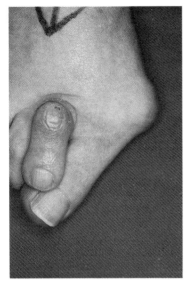 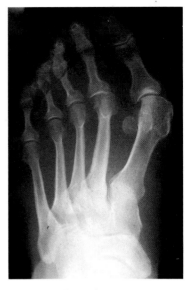

Fig. 204 Hallux valgus. Note the deformity of the second toe.

Fig. 205 Hallux valgus.

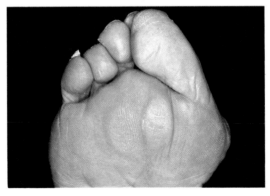

Fig. 206 Plantar callosities associated with hallux valgus.

Hallux rigidus

Osteoarthritis of the metatarsophalangeal joint of the great toe. Probably secondary to previous injury.

Clinical features

Equally common in men and women. Unlike OA in other joints, young people in their 30s are often affected.

There is discomfort in the joint, especially when the toe is dorsiflexed, e.g. when 'toeing-off' from the ground during walking.

On examination there is often a visible dorsomedial osteophyte, over which a bursa may form (Fig. 207). Passive dorsiflexion of the joint is limited (Fig. 209).

Radiographs show typical changes of OA, with narrowing of joint space, osteophytes and sclerosis of subchondral bone (Fig. 208).

Treatment

Conservative. Comfortable shoes. A bar on the sole of the shoe under the metatarsal heads will prevent painful dorsiflexion of the great toe but is rather clumsy in practice.

Surgical. For severe symptoms only. Recommended operations are arthrodesis of the joint in slight dorsiflexion, or interpositional arthroplasty using a silicone rubber spacer.

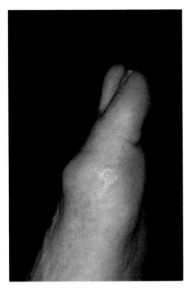

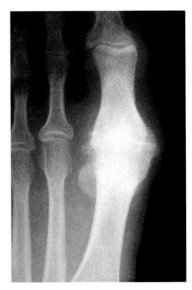

Fig. 207 Hallux rigidus. Flexion deformity and dorsal osteophyte.

Fig. 208 Radiographic appearance of hallux rigidus.

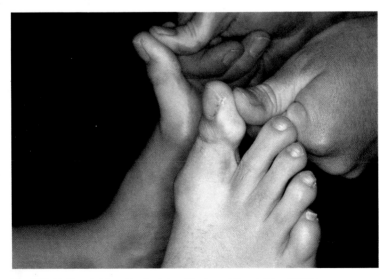

Fig. 209 Hallux rigidus. Limited dorsiflexion of the right great toe.

Bunionette (tailor's bunion)

Prominence of the head of the fifth metatarsal bone. Often associated with an overlying bursa.

Clinical features

Usually bilateral (Fig. 210). Most often seen in teenaged girls. Shoe fitting may be a problem.

Treatment

Symptoms are usually relieved by wearing broadfitting shoes. Surgical treatment is rarely needed; the recommended operations are osteotomy of the neck of the fifth metatarsal bone, or excision of the metatarsal head.

Accessory bones

These are common in the foot. Generally speaking they are of no clinical significance but may be mistaken for fractures on radiographs and sometimes cause local prominences in the foot. They are usually bilateral.
Examples are:
Os trigonum. Lies behind the talus and above the calcaneum. Sometimes attached to one of these bones (Fig.211).
Os tibiale externum. Lies on the medial border of the foot in association with the navicular bone (Fig. 212). Sometimes associated with a mobile flat foot due to an abnormal insertion of the tendon of tibialis posterior.

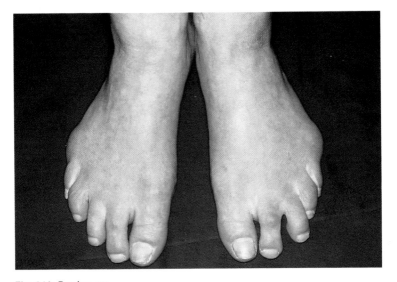

Fig. 210 Bunionette.

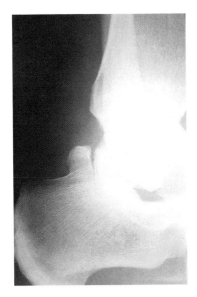

Fig. 211 An os trigonum attached to the calcaneum.

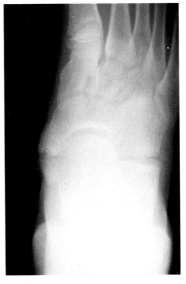

Fig. 212 Os tibiale externum.

Plantar interdigital neuroma (Morton's neuroma)

A fibrous thickening of the interdigital nerve between the third and fourth metatarsal heads. Not a true neuroma but may be due to local ischaemia or entrapment.

Clinical features

Affects middle-aged women predominantly. The complaint is of burning, neuritic pain passing into the third and fourth toes after standing or walking. Sometimes eased by taking off the shoe and rubbing the foot. Often no abnormality on clinical examination, but sometimes there is local discomfort over the site of the 'neuroma' (Fig. 213).

Treatment

A metatarsal pad may relieve the discomfort. If it does not the lesion is removed (Fig. 214). The loss of sensation between the toes causes no problems.

Plantar fibromatosis

The formation of a nodule or nodules of fibrous tissue within the plantar fascia.

This rather uncommon condition can occur in childhood or adult life. In adults it may be associated with Dupuytren's disease of the hand (p. 101) or occur as an isolated condition.

Treatment

If the lesions are large (Fig. 215) or their nature is in doubt they should be excised. Troublesome recurrence is not uncommon at any age.

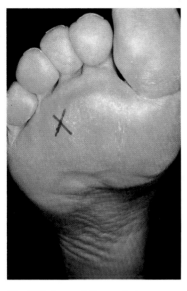

Fig. 213 Area of discomfort produced by an interdigital neuroma.

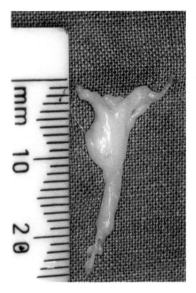

Fig. 214 An excised 'neuroma'.

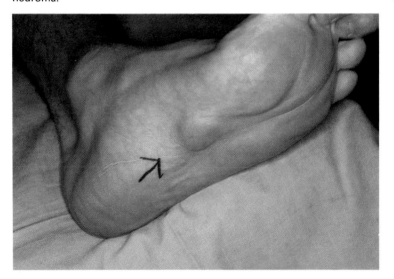

Fig. 215 Plantar fibromatosis.

Onychogryphosis

Thickened, deformed nails; usually worst on the big toe (Fig. 216). Often a result of neglect of foot care and most commonly seen in elderly people who are unable to care for themselves.

Treatment

Regular care of the nails by a chiropodist. Surgical ablation of the nail fold if regrowth is a problem.

Subungual exostosis

A bony outgrowth from the terminal phalanx of the great toe. May be associated with chronic infection around the nail. Usually affects young people.

Clinical features

The nail is raised off its bed and there is usually discomfort over the exostosis. Granulation tissue may overlie the exostosis (Fig. 217).
Radiographs show the bony prominence (Fig. 218).

Treatment

Surgical excision.

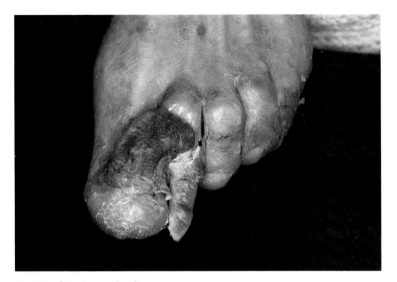

Fig. 216 Onychogryphosis.

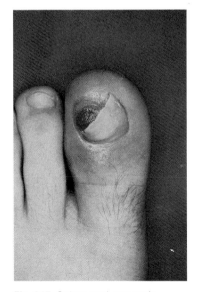

Fig. 217 Subungual exostosis.

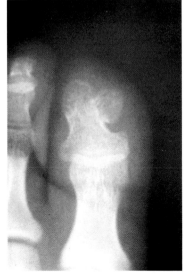

Fig. 218 Subungual exostosis.